Brass Ring Memoirs

Encouraging stories using practical methodologies
to help caregivers reach for their goals in
Alzheimer's and dementia care

Kelly McCarthy

Published by CreateSpace Independent Publishing Platform

Book cover design by MB Hebert.

Photograph on cover and in Chapter 2 by Kerry M. Hood.

Edited by Kathleen Rose.

Permission granted for cover photograph of carousel by Crescent Park, Riverside RI.

Neither the publisher nor the author is engaged in rendering professional advice or services to the individual reader. The ideas, procedures, and suggestions in this book are not intended as a substitute for consulting with a physician. All matters regarding health require medical supervision. Neither the author nor the publisher shall be liable or responsible for any loss or damage allegedly arising from any information or suggestion in this book. The reader should regularly consult a medical or behavioral professional in matters relating to his/her health, treatment, and care planning, particularly with respect to any symptoms that may require diagnosis or medical attention.

Brass Ring Memoirs uses known successful methodologies, which may not work for everyone. Caring for, or working with persons who are living with dementia is by its nature potentially dangerous. Suggested approaches and techniques should be avoided if they put you or the person in your care at any harm or risk.

While the author has made every effort to provide accurate telephone numbers and Internet addresses at the time of publication, neither the publisher nor the author assumes any responsibility for errors or changes that occur after publication. Further, the publisher does not have any control over and does not assume any responsibility for author or third-party websites or their content. All recommendations are for informational purposes only, and neither the author nor the publisher are responsible for any consequences that may occur if readers follow the advice.

Brass Ring Memoirs is a collection of stories and methodologies that use a person-centered approach to dementia care. In reference to specific individual examples, names have been changed to respect privacy.

Dedication

I dedicate this book to the past, present and future individuals who walk this path. My life will forever be blessed by the people I have and will continue to connect with on my journey as a caregiver. Whether I know you as; a colleague, an associate from a community, a family member, or a person challenged with memory loss, you have made an imprint on my life. I thank you for the moments we shared.

Acknowledgement

Have you ever looked at something and thought this is bigger than my capabilities? For many years the thought of this book was in my heart and on my tongue. I began writing this a dozen times only to listen to my head say for whatever reason, *you can't do this*. If this sounds familiar to any of you my advice is to start listening to someone else. Mary Beth, thank you for believing in me, for knocking down my walls, and for giving me the courage to believe in myself. I love you for being you and for showing me anything is possible.

Contents

Foreword

By Sharon Roth Maguire MS, RN, GNP-BC

Living with dementia presents extraordinary challenges not only for the individual with dementia but for those that love and care for them. Over the past 30 plus years, as an advance practice nurse specializing in elder care, an academic, and a thought leader, I have had the privilege of being part of the journey to better understand and support thousands of searching souls in this.

I have come to believe that the fundamental humanness of each of us and the understanding of that, is what makes a difference in the nature of the journey being a tolerable and potentially even positive experience versus an overwhelmingly frustrating and negative one.

I'm not saying this can be easy. Quite the contrary, the gradual but certain erosion of one's self and their cognitive, social, emotional, physical and functional abilities is one of the most difficult and gut wrenching experiences one can have to endure or observe.

But individuals with dementia have not lost their fundamental humanness, and though often deeply hidden and little understood, *it is there and it remains*. Joy, beauty, dignity, connection, and purpose can still exist for them when we acknowledge and honor their humanness, their individuality, their "Hazelness of Hazel." Equally importantly, when we acknowledge and honor our own humanness and reach out for the help and support we need as the care partners of persons living with dementia.

Kelly McCarthy's book, Brass Rings Memoir helps us remember that humanness, gives us tools to find it, to navigate the journey and ultimately grab that metaphorical brass ring and celebrate it. Loved ones and professionals alike will find many pearls of wisdom in Kelly's essential book. She captures well the countless trainings on dementia she has conducted as well as the individual consultations she has provided to address some of the more challenging attributes of dementia. You will feel empowered to continue the journey and will have the practical tools to make it a less overwhelming one. You will learn not only about the brass rings we all hope to grab but also about the iceberg of identity that is uniquely us and still most certainly present and relevant, perhaps even more so when we have dementia. I am honored to have reviewed and now recommend Kelly's book as an important resource for those seeking to better navigate their journey; we all have much to gain from her wisdom.

Sharon Roth Maguire, MS, RN, GNP-BC
Chief Clinical Quality Officer
BrightStar Group Holdings

Sharon oversees the BrightStar Care clinical-quality platform including operationalizing the client care experience, designing clinical operational systems for domestic and international BrightStar Care locations, and managing clinical policies and procedures. Additionally, she leads Joint Commission accreditation and related processes, clinical program development, and plays a significant role in BrightStar Senior Living, BrightStar's first residential product line focused on assisted living and memory care.

Before coming to BrightStar, Roth Maguire served as Senior Vice President of Health and Ancillary Services at Horizon Bay Retirement Living in Tampa, a senior housing company with over 90 properties in 20 states. In this role, Maguire was responsible for the oversight and execution of strategic company objectives within healthcare and memory care product lines including Medicare home health and private duty home care. Prior to Horizon Bay, Roth Maguire was the Vice President of Clinical Services for Brookdale Senior Living. A publicly traded for-profit senior care and housing company, Brookdale is the nation's largest provider of senior care with over 1000 properties in 42 states.

In addition to Maguire's extensive healthcare background, she has served on numerous boards and associations in the industry, including the Alzheimer's Association, the Assisted Living Federation of America and was the President of the National Conference of Gerontological Nurse Practitioners. She has been published in various professional and industry journals and authored chapters in well respected textbooks. She speaks at the national level on a variety of topics relevant to senior care including dementia, falls, therapeutic environments, person-centered care, and healthcare informatics. Roth Maguire has taught in both graduate and undergraduate nursing programs, most recently in the role of clinical assistant professor at Marquette University.

Introduction

Within the pages of this book are the real life stories of the people I have met along my journey as a caregiver for individuals with memory loss, and the experience and knowledge I acquired over the past 20 plus years. My journey actually began during my childhood, and it was from those early experiences that lead me on this amazing path in senior care.

The two people who influenced me the most during my childhood were my nana and my father. The positive impact they made on me truly helped in choosing a career in senior care.

My nana was not only a wonderful life mentor, she was my best friend, and I spent most of my youth with her. I held onto every word as she told me stories about her past. We had such a special bond. I was blessed to be by her side holding her hand as she took her last breath at the age of 94.

Some of my earliest memories as a child were when my father would take me with him most Sundays after church to the nursing home to visit his step-mother. As we walked along toward her room, I received a lot of attention from the residents in the hallway who smiled and said hello. For me, this place was a happy experience full of life and love.

Along with being the primary caregiver for my nana, after classes during high school I worked as a home health aide. Immediately realizing nursing wasn't for me, it was the emotional connection with people that moved me to decide on what my life's work would be. While attending college I worked in recreational therapy, and although I enjoyed it, I wanted to do more so I obtained my administrator's license and worked as a nursing home administrator for 8 years. My career path changed when my children were born, and even though I was a stay at home mom I found the time to care for seniors in a different way. My then 3 year old daughter and I would travel to nursing homes in a van full of farmyard babies, bringing the menagerie of little creatures to seniors.

After 6 years of staying at home I got back into the workforce as the director of an adult day care program, and after that I began what I knew would be my niche, the most fulfilling aspect of caregiving for me — memory care.

Throughout these many years, what I have found to be the most important has been to support the community and home-based caregivers. The family members, the friends, the front-line care associates, all those dedicated caregivers who become the voice for their loved ones and those they are caring for. It is so important to provide them with the tools they will need to be the most effective in their daily care. So along with my years of support in providing educational programs, I was asked to put together a book, a guide, in the hope of reaching many more people. When it was suggested I write a book I was honored, but a bit frightened, and as someone with dyslexia this task was the furthest thing from my mind. My learning disability never stopped me before, and although this was one obstacle I didn't think I would be able to overcome, I was up for the challenge. So, for all of you who asked, this book is for you. It is full of creative support techniques, approaches, and familiar catchphrases to support you in caring for those with memory loss.

These are real-time concepts that are intended to support you on the spot. You will learn about the global term I use, "Reaching for the Brass Ring." The Brass Ring approach will help the reader learn to recognize and understand what the aspirations are of the person you are caring for. It is also intended to assist you in identifying opportunities where you can feel safe to "let go" and focus on what the person you are caring for feels is "right" at that moment.

Next, is the Iceberg concept, and the phrase I use to show caregivers how essential a person's life story is, "What is under a person's iceberg." Readers will discover how to dive below the surface of an individual's life journey to see how to support communication and the process of how to uncover the reasons for possible challenging behaviors.

Last but not least, and my favorite concept, is the Peacock Moment. The reader will gain knowledge in the power of providing pride, beauty, and confidence for anyone. Taking the good we learn from both Reaching for the Brass Ring and what we learn under someone's iceberg, and turning it into action with peacock moments.

So, what does a Brass Ring, an Iceberg, and a Peacock have in common? Please, read on. The challenges that come with Alzheimer's disease and related dementias are not easy. I have often said I wish I had a magic wand, but we don't always get it right and sometimes the most important lesson is the one we get wrong. You must forgive yourself when you do not get things right. This book is intended to help you get back on track.

At the end of each chapter there will be takeaways for the community and home-based caregivers. No matter which type of caregiver you are, I encourage you to read both takeaways so you will appreciate and have a better understanding of what the other goes through.

I pride myself on being both a teacher and a student, so it is my hope that you learn and share the techniques and approaches within these chapters.

So, walk with me now and meet these extraordinary people whose experiences will make you laugh, cry, and learn.

CHAPTER 1
Take Care of Yourself

"Put your own mask on first."
Flight Attendant

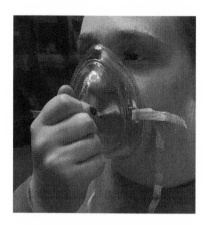

All of the chapters within this book are intended to assist you as a caregiver, whatever your capacity, and although I initially struggled with where to place this topic, I realized it is the first thing you must do.

For about seven years I traveled by plane every week, sometimes taking multiple plane rides in one week. Many of my fellow passengers would talk right through the flight attendant's announcements.

CHAPTER 1

I must admit that during some of the announcements my attention would fall off as well. But, there was one announcement that I paid close attention to. I liked it so much that I use it often when I speak at a caregivers' program. Regardless of the airline, the flight attendant would say something like, "Put your own mask on first before assisting the person next to you." To me, this is so important with caregiving, and the bottom line is, you are no good to the person you are caring for if you don't take care of yourself first.

Joe and Patty's Story

For many years I facilitated family support groups for a local Alzheimer's chapter. One group in particular stands out — it was here that I met Joe.

Joe was a retired engineer who was now struggling with the daily care tasks of being the sole caregiver for his wife, Patty, who had Alzheimer's disease. Joe and Patty were married for more than 60 years, and he had always been her knight in shining armor.

CHAPTER 1

Like many caregivers, Joe watched his wife slowly lose not only memories, but judgment related to tasks she once found very easy to complete. This was difficult for Joe, and he once said to me it was like losing half of himself.

Joe admitted that his greatest struggle was seeing his wife fail and how he desperately wanted her to be right. He said, "I constantly correct her and say, 'No, you're wrong!', and I feel so bad afterward."

During one session I asked Joe, "What do you do when your wife says it is Friday when it is really Wednesday?" His eyes welled with tears as he said, "I all but tell her she's stupid." I gently asked, "What would be the disadvantage of telling her she is right, or at least not telling her she is wrong?"

Joe understood what I was getting at, but he admitted he just could not do that. From Joe's reality, Patty could only be right when she responded with the correct information.

CHAPTER 1

I asked Joe to try something. At least once a day, let your wife be "right." As long as it does not cause harm, try not to correct her. The following week Joe came back to the group session and said to me, "I think you are onto something."

Imagine waking up every day and correcting a person who is wrong many times during the day. Why do you think Joe and many others like him have trouble with this? What toll do you think this can take on a caregiver or the person with memory loss?

A four year study suggests that being a caregiver who is experiencing mental or emotional strain is an independent risk factor for mortality among elderly spousal caregivers.[1]

Caregivers who report stress associated with caregiving are more likely to die sooner than non-caregivers.

This chapter is not meant to scare you. This is important, factual information about you as a caregiver. All too often we as caregivers like to think

CHAPTER 1

we are invincible. Caregiver stress is real, and I have seen firsthand the toll it takes on people.

This disease is tough. It takes away so much of what the individual has learned and loves.

One very difficult part of caring for people with a disease that causes dementia is the fact that we, by nature, have been programmed to live in our own reality, identifying what is right and wrong, good and bad.

All our lives, from day one as children, many of us were taught right from wrong, good from bad, and never to lie. Although we fail sometimes, for most of us this has always been what we strive for in life. The person with memory loss feels exactly the same way, so here is when the tug of war begins. They think they are right, and you want them to be right.

The challenge with this disease as a caregiver is that through our own understanding of what is right and wrong, it may become a knee-jerk reaction to correct those with memory loss to maintain our own state of being right. Some caregivers do very well

CHAPTER 1

with letting go of the things that are not always correct, and some find this extremely challenging.

Constantly correcting a person with memory loss may not only negatively affect them, but you as well. Do you see how this can create a platform for an argument or other emotional response? One way a person with memory loss may respond is with sadness at constantly being corrected, which can spiral into depression.

Let's return to Joe and Patty. He continued to attend the support group for many months. Joe was a wonderfully dedicated husband who wanted to take care of his wife. "Til death do us part" meant everything to him. He still struggled with correcting his wife and wanted her to be right. He was in a sense, programmed, because he was so used to being on the same wavelength as his wife. We have heard couples say they have been together for so long they are able to complete each other's sentences, and this was the same for Joe and Patty prior to the disease. Joe just could not fathom the loss of who he knew Patty to be for all those years.

CHAPTER 1

She was slowly disappearing right in front of his eyes.

Sadly, Joe predeceased his wife. I was working as the director of a local memory care neighborhood and received a frantic call from Patty's son, who told me what happened and asked if we could conduct an emergency admission for Patty.

Fortunately, we were able to take Patty that day, and during the screening process Patty asked multiple times, "Where is Joe?"

The family had originally shared with Patty that Joe passed away, and repeating to her that Joe died caused her upset and stress. With this particular instance, the family and I agreed on using a fiblet. We told her that Joe was with their son. A fiblet is a therapeutic white lie that decreases anxiety.[2] This is not to say that every circumstance should be dealt with by using a fiblet, but often it helps alleviate undue stress.

CHAPTER 1

I do not have the professional authority to state that this is proof that Joe's death was attributed to the stress of being a caregiver. What I do know is that Joe experienced a weekly struggle. He was in good health, was an avid golfer, and rode his bicycle throughout his town. He also belonged to a weekly men's group. But, he stopped doing all the things he enjoyed when Patty was diagnosed. Joe refused to let anyone else be responsible for his wife while he was doing something that, in his mind, was not as important as being a caregiver.

The group did try to encourage Joe to go out and do the things he enjoyed, but he felt too guilty.
Do you, or someone you know, feel the same way Joe did?

I have created the Brass Ring Oath, to support caregivers through the journey of caring for someone with memory loss. In Chapter 2 we will review in detail the Brass Ring method. The Brass Ring Oath is a pledge to yourself and is intended to remind you of the importance of putting your own mask on first.

CHAPTER I

Reaching for the Brass Ring Oath

1. I will say yes when someone offers help.
2. I will forgive myself when I do not get it right.
3. I will reach for my brass ring and I will do my best to reach for the brass ring of those I am caring for.
4. I will live in the moment, yet plan for the future.
5. I will find moments in the day to self-reflect and not feel selfish in the process.
6. I will pay attention to my health and follow up on challenges right away.
7. I will provide and accept peacock moments, which create pride, beauty, and confidence.
8. I will laugh appropriately in public and give myself permission to laugh in private, maintaining respect and dignity for the person I am caring for.
9. I will respectfully share what is under the person's iceberg to support the caregivers who are helping me.
10. I will draw strength from what I deem to be my belief system.

CHAPTER 1

Work-Life Balance

I am honored to be facilitating a virtual support group for family caregivers of young onset Alzheimer's and other related dementias, and one of the common topics is work-life balance. The above Brass Ring Oath can be the foundation when working towards work-life balance. I understand this is easier said than done. It is important to find those moments for you to be as successful as possible on this journey. There is no single answer in how to create work-life balance. Instead of breaking it down to time, think of it as a moment. Try filling yourself up by grazing on those moments.

Joe's story underscores why this chapter goes first. It is very important to know that you are not shunning your responsibilities when you take care of yourself and put systems in place to help support you. This is how you create a balance between taking care of yourself and taking care of someone else.

CHAPTER 1

It is never too late to ask for help, and there are other support references in the endnotes of this book. The following are just a few national support programs that have local support services all over the country:

Alzheimer's Association
225 N Michigan Ave
Chicago, IL 60611-7633
24/7 Helpline 1-800-272-3900
www.alz.org

Alzheimer's Foundation of America
322 Eighth Avenue, 7th floor
New York, NY 10001
Helpline 1-866-232-8484
www.alzfdn.org

CHAPTER 1

The Takeaway

For home-based caregivers: When someone asks, "Do you want help?" don't even give it a second thought. Just say "yes!" You may not know what you need help with at the moment, but you can figure it out later. Sometimes the hardest thing is to accept help, so rip it off like a bandage and say yes!

For community caregivers: Choosing to work in memory care is a noble vocation and like many jobs you may be asked to work extra shifts. Many communities frown upon routinely staffing double shifts. Consistently putting in long hours every week may increase stress, causing you to not be at your best, which may result in frustration toward the people you are caring for. Make sure to check in to make sure you are taking care of yourself. Just like the home-based caregivers, you need to pay attention to work-life balance

Chapter 2

Reaching for the Brass Ring

"We need to care as much about preventing broken spirits as we do about preventing broken limbs."
Rabbi Sam Seicol

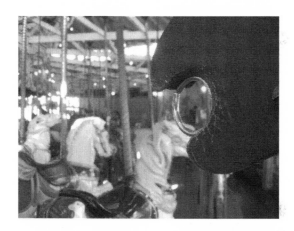

As the music begins and the wooden dobby horses start to move ever so slowly up and down, the children gaze at their parents with bright, gleaming eyes. The carousel turns faster and the children's hearts flutter with anticipation. Then the moment finally arrives. It is time to reach for the brass ring! Currently there are only 11 operational brass ring game carousels left in the USA[1] and one of them is

Chapter 2

the Crescent Park Carousel in Riverside, Rhode Island, which was the backdrop for the cover of this book. The carousel is still operational and open to visitors.

The concept of the carousel game is to find and obtain the brass rings. Children of all ages climb up onto colorfully decorated wooden horses that are attached to a large merry-go-round. On the outer edge of the carousel there is a long arm that dispenses rings and is suspended just within reach of those on the horses. Interspersed among the steel or iron rings is one brass ring.

It is important to pull all the other rings out of the arm in the hope that a brass ring will fall in its place. If you are lucky enough to grab the brass ring the prize is a free ride, but the glory of the brass ring is so much more rewarding than being able to ride again for free. Reaching for the "brass ring" does not end as you age. Take a moment to identify the brass rings in your life such as graduating from college or finding that fantastic job. How about asking for a divorce? Brass rings are not always happy moments

CHAPTER 2

in our lives and sometimes they are a part of a difficult journey.

As we go through life, our brass ring changes. We either accomplish our intended goal or surrender and move on to the next new possible feat. What we reach for and get, and what we reach for and don't get, all contribute to who we are as individuals. The good news is the sun still comes up even though we do not obtain some of the brass rings we are reaching for.

I use the brass ring as a metaphor in caring for people with memory loss. Now let's think about this concept in caregiver's terms. As the disease progresses, individuals with memory challenges may forget what their "brass rings" were, and knowing their life's journey can assist you in reaching for their brass ring as a caregiver, a loving family member, or a friend.

When you are caring for someone with memory loss you should think about short term brass rings and

CHAPTER 2

long term brass rings for both the individual you are caring for and for yourself as caregiver. For example, as the caregiver, your short term goal may be to get the person up and showered, dressed, fed their breakfast, and be on time for an appointment. Sometimes we as caregivers are holding on, white knuckled to our brass ring. We hold on so tight to the "task" that we lose sight of the person.

Your loved one may want everything you are reaching for except the shower! What do we do then? Well, this is when you consider dropping your brass ring and picking up theirs. Caring for someone with this disease is not easy. Give yourself and the one you are caring for a break.

Many times I have heard caregivers say, "I have to give her a shower!" Remember, that is not their brass ring and you are trying to force them to reach for yours. You may have an argument or even a physical altercation on your hands as a result. When a person with memory loss is upset with you or the circumstance surrounding a shower, you must let it go and try again later. Never force someone into the

CHAPTER 2

shower or use multiple people to assist while the person with memory loss is kicking and screaming. How would you feel if that were you?

The first thing is to know what your brass ring is in caring for someone with memory loss and understanding when the person you are caring for does not have the same brass rings you do. Have no fear, it is not the end of the world, and later in the book we will discuss other ways to help support both yourself as caregiver and the person with memory loss in achieving brass rings.

We have already talked about short term brass rings, so let's talk about long term brass rings. Long term brass rings go in two different directions. Caregivers' long term goals go forward, such as financial planning, family support, and outside services. When we talk about long term brass rings for individuals with memory loss, the direction changes and goes backwards. For example, a man challenged with memory loss may be extremely proud when you recognize him for serving our country. A woman who had a successful business may love talking about being a woman in a time

CHAPTER 2

when the workforce was dominated by men. Knowing what their long term brass rings were helps us stay connected.

It can be just as important to know the brass rings that were missed and how you as a caregiver can support the individual. This may also be a sore spot for them and may want to be avoided, as it may trigger an upset or create a depressing mood. For example, someone never got married so instead, they sacrificed and took care of their parents in their old age. The road not taken can be a difficult road to bear and even tougher if it is stuck in the person's long term memory as a missed brass ring. Honor the person's feelings and let them know you care. As we do with a friend, we must let them vent even though we do not have answers. It is still good to allow them to express their feelings. Tell them it is okay to feel down about the road not taken, and how wonderful that this journey she has been on led her straight to you! Don't be afraid to let people sit where they need to sit, then share the silver lining.

CHAPTER 2

Three things to consider while reading this book:

1. We all have brass rings. As a caregiver you need to know when to let yours go. Even though you are holding on tight, it is important to honor the person you are caring for by picking up their brass ring.
2. Congratulations! If you are reading this book you are now officially reaching for a new brass ring.
3. This is not easy. Remember, you are wonderful and although you may not always get it right, you are not alone. Forgive yourself.

Sally - "Is This the Old Carriage House?"

I was the director of a memory care neighborhood that just opened and Sally was one of our first residents. I bet Sally never thought she would make such an impact on me.

CHAPTER 2

Sally was a high functioning woman, both physically and cognitively, with a great sense of humor. She loved the actor Robert Taylor. She said she even met him once at a local naval base. One of her favorite sayings was, "Such is life without a wife and here I am without a man." Sally was a wonderful woman who taught me so much about memory loss.

The first thing Sally taught me was a lesson in the act of repeating. Not every day, but often, Sally would ask a question not just once, not just twice, but many times. As students we look for the unmet need. Are they lonely, tired, hungry, or in pain? Perhaps they are bored.

With Sally it didn't seem to be any of these. There was something else. When Sally was experiencing one of her moments of repetition she would ask, "Is this the old Carriage House?" When Sally asked this once we knew there was a likelihood of her asking us many times. This repetition is an example of Sally having a moment of lucidity. When she made the connection it stuck with her throughout the day. She was most likely saying, I know where I am, and she was right! This new community was indeed once a restaurant and function hall called The Carriage House.

So please, be sensitive. Even though we may hear someone ask a question many times, which can be frustrating for us, it is important to remember the person with memory loss is being robbed of the ability to remember and to them are only asking the question once.

One day I was walking through the dining room and noticed Sally gazing out the window. She seemed to be looking down the road, and when I approached her she asked, "Is this the old Carriage House?" I said, "Yes this is the old Carriage House and I used to come here for dinner and sometimes even for a wedding." Sally smiled and said, "Me too!"

"Is that so?", I replied. A few minutes later Sally asked, "Is this the old Carriage House?" I said, "Yes this is the old Carriage House, and you used to come here for weddings, didn't you?" She replied, "Yes, I did come here for weddings and I even ate at the restaurant a couple of times."

Chapter 2

As she continued to look out the window Sally said, "I used to live down the road a bit." Seconds later she looked back into the dining room and asked, "Is this the old Carriage House?"

I again responded, "Yes, Sally, it is the old Carriage House. Didn't you live down the road a bit?" Sally said, "I did! 133 Stanton Street." I said, "Well that's right down there," and as she returned her gaze toward the window and down the road she said, "Yes, right down there I used to live on 133 Stanton Street with my daughter and son for many years. Our backyard was near the bay. It was a relatively small yard, but because we were near the bay, my kids said we had the biggest yard in the world." We both laughed at that and I agreed how great it must have been to grow up enjoying the shore.

What Sally taught me was to not only respect the person and answer them like it was the first time they asked the question, but to stop, listen, and take the time to learn. Sally was showing me her moments of lucidity, her brass ring, and that raising those children in such a lovely place was her peacock moment (defined in Chapter 4) for remembering what once was. If I simply said "Yes, this is the old Carriage House, Sally" and walked away, I would not have been blessed to know what I learned about my dear friend.

Although Sally taught me something that only took one day to learn, she was not done teaching me. Within that year I was promoted to memory care specialist and began flying all over the country supporting other communities. Sally's community was still mine to oversee in a regional capacity and to visit periodically, and after about a year into my new position I made a routine visit back to the old Carriage House.

During my visit the program director shared with me that Sally's health had declined and that she was no longer able to speak, but she would most likely enjoy a visit just the same. She had been moved to the health center area of the building and as I approached her room I knocked and entered. Sally's eyes were wide open and once again she was staring out the window just as she had done a year ago. I sat by Sally's bed and gently reached over placing my hand in hers, and for a brief moment I thought to

CHAPTER 2

myself, "How am I going to communicate with you now?" Without a word she turned and looked at me and I knew exactly what to do.

"Hey Sally, it's Kelly. This is the old Carriage House and you and I used to come here for weddings and even ate here at the restaurant." As Sally looked at me, and while caressing her hands I continued, "You used to live right down the road at 133 Stanton Street, and your kids were so lucky they would always say they had the best backyard in the world."

My visit with Sally ended as it always had, and I gave her a kiss and recited her favorite saying, "Such is life without a wife and here I am without a man." It was such a blessing for me to know Sally and what I learned from her. Her second lesson was, even though we don't know where the person we are caring for is at in their journey, and in their ability to comprehend what is being said, I was able to communicate to her the stories that were so dear to her life. The story — her story — was familiar. She was calm and although not oriented, she was alert and seemed to enjoy the time we spent together. That's the goal you are looking for as a caregiver or when visiting your loved ones. You want the connection to either be familiar, loving or both. You do not need to get a verbal response from them to know you have made an impression. As I held Sally's hand, she didn't say anything, but the words she once spoke were the same words I was now speaking for her, and that makes all the difference.

The Takeaway

For home-based caregivers: As caregiver you have goals for the immediate moment, the day, the week. Those goals may be different than the goals of the person you are caring for. We have brass rings and they have brass rings. Appreciate and understand that when someone is not in any danger, you may just want to put your brass ring down and pick their brass ring up.

For community caregivers: You are working in the community and you have tasks to accomplish. Those are your brass rings. Stop, listen, and take the time to learn. Knowing a person's brass ring prior to care can make them feel connected and valued by you. It is not just about the activities of daily living

CHAPTER 2

(ADL) care. It is very important to find a balance between connecting with the person you are caring for and doing the tasks.

CHAPTER 3
The Iceberg

"Look beneath the surface; let not the several quality of a thing nor its worth escape thee."
Marcus Aurelius

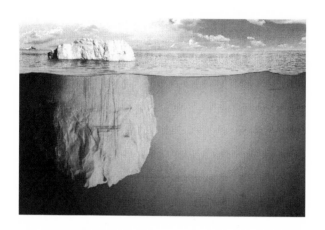

If you are a home-based caregiver of a loved one with memory loss you have an initial advantage over an outside agency or community caregiver simply because you know the person. However, that does not imply you should be the only person who can or should care for your loved one. It is important for all caregivers to learn as much as possible about the person they are caring for.

CHAPTER 3

Imagine caring for someone with memory loss over a period of time and not knowing anything about them but their diagnosis. When you try asking them questions about who they are, they have difficulty answering and you have only a diagnosis to work with and not the person.

Our self-identity is celebrated and reinforced through the relationships we have. I can say I am an educator all day long, but it is my profession and experience that reinforces this when I teach. If I had no one to teach, I would no longer be able to validate my identity as an educator.

Individuals with memory challenges progressively lose their sense of self. You as the caregiver can maintain their sense of self by honoring who the person is through their life experiences. During my trainings I often talk about the "iceberg" when referring to how we get to know someone. After listening to me for only a few moments, I would ask the group of caregivers what they know about me. Here is what they usually say:

CHAPTER 3

- Your name is Kelly.
- You teach memory care and travel for a living.
- You wear glasses.
- You have a sense of humor and are passionate about what you do.

Do you think having this information is enough if you are going to care for me? A caregiver must know more than what is on the top of the iceberg to be actively and successfully engaged in an individual's care.

Knowing basic information about a person works for individuals without memory loss because a caregiver is able to engage in conversation about likes and dislikes, brass rings, etc. Some individuals with memory loss in early stages can give you a history, but knowing that Alzheimer's and many other related dementias are progressive, it is crucial to learn what we can about someone early on. What is below the iceberg? You should know the good, the bad, and the ugly, and you still need to share. You should know, not to judge, but to honor and know what to talk about and what not to talk about.

CHAPTER 3

When you meet someone for the first time what do you know about them?

How about if you chat with them for an hour, what do you learn?

Iceberg Exercise:

I encourage you to draw an iceberg similar to the one shown here.

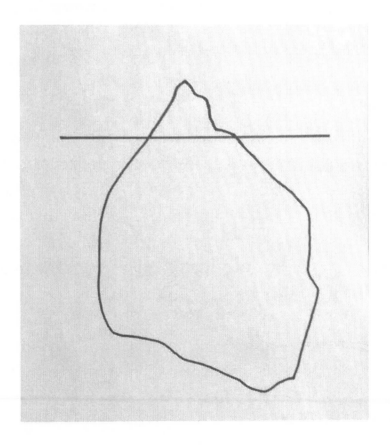

CHAPTER 3

Using the person with memory loss, begin by identifying what you see and what you hear from the person and placing that on the top. Next, fill out the bottom of the iceberg with things that are not visible yet essential for successfully building a connection with the individual. Some examples are: faith, family, hobbies, music, medical history, personality, education, and sexuality, to name a few. One of the areas I have seen be so impactful is the knowledge of how to connect through music. Music, for many truly touches the soul. Reconnecting with past musical favorites can often create a successful emotional connection. I was fortunate to meet one of the founders of Music and Memory© during a conference in Wisconsin Dells. It was amazing to see the impact personal music preferences had on many individuals in all stages of Alzheimer's and related dementias. The following link is from Music and Memory© and is a wonderful example of the impact this program had on a man named Henry. https://www.youtube.com/watch?v=5FWn4JB2YLU

The Iceberg is different from the Brass Ring. The Iceberg is the action of learning who the person is. This is where you learn what the person's Brass

CHAPTER 3

Rings are and what makes a peacock moment (more to come on peacock moments in Chapter 4). It is the act of discovery. With the Iceberg concept you will be diving deep under the surface to discover a person's likes, dislikes, personality traits, and triggers to avoid when providing care. The old saying that you are only as strong as your weakest link is a very important statement when referring to the team of caregivers. So, whether there are only two caregivers or twenty two, **<u>everyone</u>** needs to discover as much as possible about the person they are caring for and how to connect with them.

When I hear a caregiver say, "I am the only one who can give 'Millie' a shower," I like to find out the why behind this. Often it can be a simple approach the caregiver is using that may be easily duplicated by others. Be open-minded to different approaches. Your success at engagement and connection may be the most important things to learn. As a caregiver it is also essential to know what **<u>not</u>** to do or say that may cause upset. It is very important for you to understand the more information you share with other caregivers the more successful the person who is challenged with memory loss will be. The pitfall to the iceberg concept is that some families may keep things private when divulging the history of their loved one because they are embarrassed, and may feel that their loved one will be judged. Please know this is not the first time an agency or community has heard the types of challenges you are faced with individually. Sharing all of what is under the iceberg is crucial for caregivers so they will know how to be successful with your loved one. It is not always easy to share information that may be uncomfortable to discuss.

Flowy - "Where's the Baby?"

"Where's the baby?"

Flowy, a resident of our memory care community kept asking this question. I talked with her husband and daughter and asked them if they knew what she meant. They were both just as perplexed as we were. I shared with them that I scoured the information in her social history that the family provided upon admission, but was not able to find anything about a baby. Flowy's daughter acknowledged that she recently heard her mother ask the same question

CHAPTER 3

and at first was just as stumped as we were until we discussed the possibility of a past situation that may be causing her to talk about a baby.

As we talked, Flowy's daughter shared that although her mom had kids, she was never really interested in children and was always timid around babies. The daughter said, "Come to think of it, she would watch my children but did not want them to sleep overnight."

Then a light bulb came on and the daughter turned to her father and said, "Dad, didn't you and mom have a SIDS[1] baby before Jack and I were born?" The father's eyes widened as he remembered, "Yes, we did."

After speaking with Flowy's husband and daughter about this being the possible "unmet" need, I shared an approach that I would take full responsibility in conducting.

I explained to the family that Flowy's life timeline was working its way back through her life. She was a mother and the art of nurturing was familiar to her.

CHAPTER 3

So, in this situation, the introduction of a life-like doll may or may not work in comforting Flowy. She was becoming increasingly distressed about the baby and having a plan to decrease her anxiety without using medication was our first priority.

Flowy was asking for the baby and there was only one way to find out if giving her the "baby" would work. Luckily my daughter was very willing to offer up one of her dolls, and we chose one with special features. The eyes opened and closed, which was helpful because we did not want Flowy to think the baby was dead, and the joints were movable.

We swaddled the doll in a baby blanket and placed a baby cap on its head and I brought it to work not knowing what the outcome would be. I was hopeful that I could make a positive difference with Flowy's request.

Before I introduced the baby to Flowy, I explained to the family what I was going to do. I told them I would be reviewing Flowy's emotional response to the baby doll at the initial introduction and throughout the day.

CHAPTER 3

I explained that I would not tell her this was her baby and just provide a general introduction. I would watch for any signs of her being overwhelmed throughout the process.

Flowy was a mid-80 year old woman with stage 5 memory loss on the Global Deterioration Scale (GDS).[2] It is very important to understand that you will not be able to introduce a doll as a baby to every stage because the earlier stages will recognize the "baby" to be a doll and think you are crazy!

It was time for me to visit Flowy. "Knock, knock! Good morning Flowy," I said as I entered her room. "Well, hello there," she replied. I cradled the doll in my arms and knelt down beside her and said, "Flowy, look who I have." Flowy looked at the "baby" and with her eyes opening wide said, "You have him! May I?" "Yes you may," and I gently handed the doll to her as she took it in her arms and said, "Here he is, here is Joey." Joey was the name of their son who died of SIDS in the 1940s.

Many things are hidden under the iceberg. Not everything is shared right away. We are not always

CHAPTER 3

proud of everything that is under there. When Flowy and her husband experienced the loss of their first child in the 1940s, SIDS was not fully understood and mothers were often accused of abuse and were interrogated.

The fathers of the children were not initially under suspicion due to the gender roles during this time period. The husband was the breadwinner and the wife took care of the house and children.

This was a traumatic moment in Flowy's mind and the baby doll comforted her and gave her peace. I called her husband and shared how she was responding to the doll. He came in later that day and saw his wife sitting in the rocking chair in her room holding the doll. He stood just outside the room and wept, and as I walked over to him he looked at me and said, "I'm not crying because my wife is holding a doll. I'm crying because she has Joey back. This disease took one away and brought another back."

Some families are not as receptive to introducing artificial items such as dolls, stuffed animals, etc., so

I do ask that you be open-minded to what makes the person feel whole again. Remember, this disease robs them of so much. Look at where the person is within the disease process and go on what you know about them to see what challenges they may be working through.

The Takeaway

For home-based caregivers: The more information you share with the support caregivers you entrust to care for your loved one, the more successful your loved one will be. Support services need your help in caring for someone you know with memory loss. This is particularly important when a residential community or home agency is assisting you in caring for your loved one. The more caregivers know what is under your loved one's iceberg, the more successful your loved one will be. Reveal everything you know and don't be embarrassed by a loved one's habit or something they may say or do. If the caregiver has specialized training in caring for those with memory loss, they will understand. They have most likely seen similar

CHAPTER 3

challenges before and they are there to support the success of your loved one.

For community caregivers: Work with the care team. Often times if the caregiver doesn't know the person they may resort to prescription medications, such as mood stabilizers, to mask the unmet need instead of initially asking what is under the person's iceberg.

Each community or agency should have a system in place to know the individual's social history. It is important to read the information and learn about the person. Even though we may be different from them, we should never judge what we find under their iceberg because we too have the good, the bad, and the ugly under ours.

If you look at the social history and don't see what you are looking for, reach out to the family or primary caregiver. Like the iceberg, approximately 90% of who we are is underneath the surface. Don't be afraid to reach out to family and work with them. You may need to jog their memory about something from the past that may be triggering a behavior.

CHAPTER 4
Peacock Moment

"Be happy in the moment, that's enough. Each moment is all we need, not more."   Mother Teresa

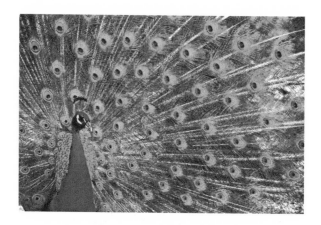

For the past 10 years I have used the visual of a peacock with its feathers fanned out in full display to illustrate the Peacock Moment concept. I stand before the group with a picture of a peacock on the screen and ask, "How do you think this guy feels?" The responses are unanimous. "Beautiful!" "Proud!" "Confident!"

Chapter 4

"What else does the peacock do?" I ask as I become the peacock, stretching out my arms and hands like feathers. "Do they just stand there?"

"No, they strut!" Off I go, strutting and fluttering my feathers in front of everyone so they may see how proud, how beautiful, and how confident I feel.

So often with Alzheimer's and other diseases with dementia related symptoms, as the disease progresses, the person is robbed of their confidence, pride, and beauty. It was this moment of realization that I began using the peacock concept to inspire caregivers to self-reflect on their communication skills.

It can be difficult to communicate positively with those who not only experience memory loss, but whose capacity to use good judgment may also be impaired and their safety is at risk.

You may realize after the fact that what you said or did was not a peacock moment. Words and phrases such as, "Stop," "No," "I told you already," "You forgot," "Don't you remember?" do not create a peacock moment. If you get it wrong, don't beat yourself up. Forgive yourself and take a break. When you are ready, try again. It may be helpful during your break to think about the act of responding to a situation rather than reacting to one. Often, our initial reactions are impulsive, done quickly with little thought, and are usually related out of our emotions at that time. We need to try to be more mindful when responding to a situation. Taking a minute to think about a reply helps us communicate in a more loving way. This will help you to create a peacock moment.

What I find that helps with this process is to find peacock moments often and not just when you are frustrated. When you are used to giving random peacock moments it becomes easier to communicate in a positive way during those times when you are a bit exasperated.

A peacock moment has proven to create positive self-reflection and helps caregivers to easily identify what to say and how to say it. This disease can be challenging for the person struggling with memory loss as well as the family and caregiver. Peacock

CHAPTER 4

moments help to instill in everyone involved that "moments" are precious in memory care.

Bob - A Proud Veteran

During one of my many visits to our Arizona memory care neighborhood, I recall a visit in particular that became a teaching moment for me.

When I arrived I met with the program director who accompanied me on my usual walk-through of the community, and he talked briefly with me about a resident named Bob.

"Kelly, I'd like you to meet someone. His name is Bob, he was a WWII veteran, and he has been having some behavior issues."

Before I could ask any further questions about Bob, the program director excused himself and said he had to take a call and that he would meet up with me afterward. As I continued on alone and was nearing the dining room I heard someone ask for help. I entered the dining room and saw a resident sitting at a table with her back to the wall and she was calmly, but loudly saying, "Help, help." The

CHAPTER 4

woman did not appear to be in distress, however, as I got closer I noticed another resident, a small man about 5'-2" who had abandoned his walker, and was pushing the small square dining room table towards this woman.

It looked to me as though the man was upset with the woman calling out for help and he was trying to say to her, "Stop yelling," in the only way he knew how. I had no idea who this man was, but I thought perhaps it could be Bob, so the first thing I did was to try and redirect him.

"Bob is that you?"

He stopped pushing the table and turned to me. I continued on with what I knew about him.

"Are you that WWII veteran I keep hearing about?" Bob was no longer holding onto the table at this point and he lifted up his left short sleeve then his right exposing a WWII tattoo on one arm, and a Merchant Marine tattoo on the other. As I put my hand out to thank him for serving our country he looked as though he grew from 5'-2" to 7 feet tall!

CHAPTER 4

Bob just taught me how to create a peacock moment for him.

Just knowing a little bit of this gentleman's brass ring allowed me to redirect and rechannel him right away. To redirect by using his name, and to rechannel by honoring him with a peacock moment, "Are you the WWII veteran I keep hearing about?" and "Thank you for your service."

Not having much information about what was under Bob's iceberg was not easy, but fortunately it was enough.

It is all too easy to use the words, "No," "Stop,'" "Don't," "Behave yourself."
The peacock moment is meant to help the caregiver by providing a way to redirect and rechannel a behavior through positive communication.

For Bob, who had about a 30 second memory recall, would not remember the event. From a good or bad encounter Bob would ride the wave of feeling proud, angry, or depressed, but would not understand the specifics as to why he was feeling that way.

66

CHAPTER 4

Many times it is only the caregiver who stays frustrated or angry, and can become resentful of a moment that is already gone from the mind of the person with memory loss.

The next chance you get, work on the peacock moment and maybe you too will see the beauty, pride, and confidence you give back to the person with memory loss.

What a gift it is!

During one of my visits to Dallas, Texas I addressed a group of caregivers and asked, "How many times would you say the residents are wrong on any given day?" A gentleman in the front row raised his hand and as I called on him he said, "Well Miss Kelly, I would say they're wrong about eight times out of ten." I asked him, "What is your goal then as a caregiver in this community?" Without hesitating he said, "It is to make them right ten times out of ten." He got it.

Chapter 4
The Takeaway

For both takeaways we must be sure the individual with memory loss is not causing harm to themselves or others in our endeavor to make them right. If this is the case, there has to be other interventions. If they are safe, walk away and give them time. (There is more on this subject in Chapter 10 - Behaviors.)

For home-based caregivers: It is difficult enough when people without disease-related dementia have disagreements. Memory loss makes it even more so. The person you may have bantered with before and have known to be right many times is now sliding into being wrong more often. You constantly win the argument but you do not feel good about it. You want them to be right. Make the person you are caring for right ten times out of ten. This disease is not easy, especially when it is you that begins to disappear in their mind. Hang in there and keep thinking about the peacock moments. Keep thinking about how you can make the person you are caring for feel beautiful, proud, and confident, even when they are wrong. At the end of the day it will be you who did it right. It is important to remember to not only give peacock moments, but to receive them.

For community caregivers:

Make the person you are caring for right ten times out of ten. This is what I feel we are sometimes missing as we go on, day after day, caring for someone with this disease who is robbed of their beauty, pride, and confidence. It is not easy, but once you get it and practice this, you find joy in each moment. Your goal as caregiver is to create many peacock moments. It is important to remember to not only give peacock moments, but to receive them.

CHAPTER 5

The Difference Between Alzheimer's and Dementia

"The person with dementia is not giving you a hard time, the person with dementia is having a hard time"
Anonymous

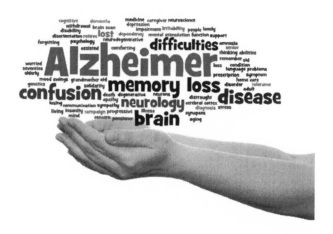

Now that we have reviewed the real-time concepts — Brass Ring, Iceberg, and Peacock Moment — which are intended to support you through caring for a person with memory loss, let's back up and review a question that we in this field are often

CHAPTER 5

asked. What is the difference between Alzheimer's and dementia?

Often in my travels I find this to be one of the most asked questions from professional caregivers and family members. A daughter once said to me, "My mother doesn't have Alzheimer's she just has dementia."

My intent of this chapter is not to concentrate on the clinical aspects of the diseases that cause dementia, but to answer the question that is asked the most in the hope that you will gain a clear understanding of what dementia is and what it is not.

I spoke with a daughter who attended an open house at an assisted living community. After the presentation she told me how much she wished she had participated in these programs sooner to have the tools she needed during some tough times with her mom. I asked her to tell me more about what she felt she needed as a resource. She explained that because her mother was not diagnosed with Alzheimer's she did not think to reach out to the Alzheimer's organization for support. She

CHAPTER 5

admittedly said she was afraid of the stigma that went along with Alzheimer's, and words like "memory loss" and "dementia" somehow lightened the diagnosis.

This daughter is not alone, and many caregivers take on the challenges of memory care without help because of the negative stereotypes that may go along with these diseases.

Many organizations that support Alzheimer's disease now also include the words "and related dementias" so that caregivers have a place of support when the diagnosis involves memory loss.

So, let me provide a brief definition for Alzheimer's disease and dementia. Please note, for a more clinical definition please see the Endnotes at the back of this book for some additional resources.

Dementia is a symptom.[1] I have worked with memory care organizations from across the country that have supported the fact that although many people, including individuals in the medical profession, have been known to use the word

CHAPTER 5

dementia synonymous with disease, it is in fact a symptom and should be clearly identified as such.

Dementia is a general term for a decline in mental ability severe enough to interfere with daily life.[2]

Alzheimer's disease is an irreversible, progressive brain disorder that slowly destroys memory and thinking skills and, eventually, the ability to carry out the simplest tasks.[3]

Some common diseases that have symptoms of dementia are, Alzheimer's, vascular dementia, and Lewy Body disease. Alzheimer's gets top billing because it is the most commonly diagnosed and accounts for approximately 60%-80% of all dementia.[4]

This book is not intended to help diagnose or go into specifics of each disease as there are currently over 100 diseases that cause the symptoms of dementia, but it is important to work with the individual's physician to identify what disease may be causing the cognitive decline. Different diseases have other symptoms that are important for you as the caregiver to know about. For example, Lewy Body disease can also have symptoms of paranoid ideations and can cause the person to have an unsteady gait.

The majority of individuals with symptoms of dementia have a progressive decline. Some signs and symptoms of a decline show more quickly than others. However, one point I would like to note is, not all signs and symptoms of decline are a result of memory loss.

Clear as mud? Hang on, I will attempt to clear this up.

There are medical conditions that can mimic the signs and symptoms of dementia. One is known as delirium. Delirium is a serious disturbance in mental abilities that results in confused thinking and reduced awareness of your environment.[5] The start of delirium is usually rapid, within hours or a few days. Some examples of when delirium would occur would be urinary tract infections (UTI) and dehydration.

CHAPTER 5

Acute confusion can also be a side effect of medication. When signs of acute confusion begin, work with the medical team to review both existing and new medication(s) as this could be the culprit.

Because symptoms of delirium and dementia can be similar, input from a family member or caregiver may be important for a doctor to make an accurate diagnosis. Why I mention this is I have often heard family members and care teams say, "Oh, her dementia is progressing," instead of ruling out other possible serious issues.

There are many other conditions that can cause delirium in older adults so it is important to connect with the individual's medical support team to rule out other medical issues that may mimic the signs of dementia.

I would like to finish this chapter about dementia by sharing a question that comes up for caregivers. The question is, "How come my dad remembers things very clearly from the past, but cannot remember what he had for lunch?"

CHAPTER 5
18 Wheeler

A simple analogy I use to help understand progressive dementia is an 18 wheeler tractor trailer. When loading the trailer, the first things in are the last out. So imagine that the 18 wheeler represents where long term memories are stored in the brain.

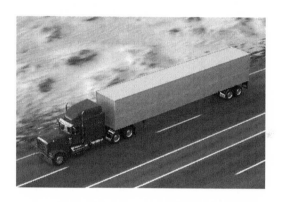

The memories that are going to be stored away safely for the longest amount of time are the foundation memories such as name, family, and faith. These memories may not have the same significance to all generations, but they are very important with the current age group we are caring for. Other examples of first memories are native language, culture/traditions, and schooling, to name a few. With these experiences come both good and bad memories. So, into the 18 wheeler they go, to the furthest part of the trailer, safe and secure.

As we go through our life's journey each memory, the good and bad, is neatly stored next to the one before it. For example, traditions, education, learning a new language, regrets from the road not taken, marriage, military service, birth of a child, divorce, remarriage, grandchildren, travel, death of a spouse, retirement, and so on.

Now the trailer is full and all of the memories are safely packed away in the order in which they have been received. The good, the bad, and the ugly ... until moving day!

Lou Asks, "Where is my wife?"

Lou was admitted to our memory care community and upon admission he was aware of and had retained the memory that his wife had passed away 10 years before. Among the other information under Lou's iceberg was the fact that his wife had been a school teacher. One year into his residency I was walking down the hallway and Lou stopped me and asked, "Where's my wife?" I was taken a bit off guard, even with my experience, as this was an abrupt change, and at this moment needed to maintain his dignity so I was able to recall what was under his iceberg. I said to him, "It's early, she may be at school," and he responded, "Oh okay, she didn't tell me where she was going."

I made a judgment call in using a fiblet to decrease Lou's anxiety regarding where his wife was. Having the information that Lou knew his wife died, it concerned me that he woke up not remembering this. The next step was working with the clinical team to rule out any medical issues that could be causing this jump in decline. The nurse called the doctor and an order for a urinalysis and blood work was given, and the results showed there was no indication of any acute medical problems.

Lou had the memory of his wife of 50 years deeply stored in his long term memory. However, the death of his wife was only 11 years old, so as a result of Lou having a diagnosis of Alzheimer's, the memory of the death of his wife was unpacked or gone before

CHAPTER 5

the memory of their married years, which resulted in him forgetting about her death.

This became Lou's new baseline — he thought his wife was still alive. Because of this we worked with the family to create individual interventions and approaches just for Lou when he asked about his wife.

Although progressive dementia can be identified as memories being lost in sequential order, as in the example of Lou's story, it should be noted that periods of lucidity can take place where the individual with memory loss can recall a moment that may have been thought to be gone.

A pitfall that may take place with caregivers when individuals with memory loss experience lucid moments is, the caregiver may think the person has been pretending. So, it is important for caregivers to understand what a lucid moment is, and to consider it is a gift when the person they are caring for gets it right. Make them feel good by giving them a peacock moment.

CHAPTER 5

Alzheimer's and other related dementias are not a part of the natural aging process, which means just because we age into our senior years, this does not mean we are going to have memory loss or disease-related dementias.

The Takeaway

For home-based caregivers: It is important for you as the caregiver/family member/friend, to honor the person and to acknowledge that although it may be very difficult to experience watching the removal of memories from their life, you being included, it is important to navigate through their timeline with them. If given the chance, honor lucidity with peacock moments. Reminiscing about the memories that you know are vivid on their timeline will assist you in making a connection.

For community caregivers: You are valued more than you know. When you notice a change in someone's baseline, it is so important for you to notify the clinical team and not just assume the person's dementia has progressed. Take a moment to review some of the ways you relay cognitive and

CHAPTER 5

physical changes of the person you are caring for. Making sure you know who to inform when a change occurs will ensure this valuable information gets passed on to the appropriate people for follow up.

CHAPTER 6
Acts of Purpose

"If I'm not being used, I'm useless."
My mom

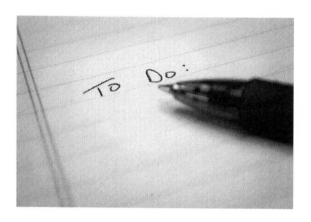

Unfortunately I would never hear my kids say, "Hey mom, give me something to do, I need to feel useful!" although I did hear my son say to my mother, "Nana, I know how much you want to feel useful, so can you take me to Game Stop?"

Both of my parents are in their 80s and find the golden years are not so golden. Besides slowing down and the ongoing aches and pains, the other pill that is difficult to swallow is the loss of purpose.

CHAPTER 6

My mom and dad have said many times, "I need to feel useful."

One of my parent's brass rings is to maintain acts of purpose. They are not alone. Many older adults find themselves in the same dilemma and are still seeking purpose well into their senior years.

Purpose helps maintain a person's identity. The tasks we perform as a parent, spouse, friend, gardener, writer, gives us all a sense of purpose. When we lose the purposeful task, we lose some of our identity.

I recently watched a video of a woman who hated the weekends because her senior center was not open. She spent the weekends opening and shredding her mail just to have something to do. I believe this is something I would have never fully understood if I were not in the industry of senior care.

People with memory loss have the same challenges we do. They often strive for purpose and we as caregivers take away what little purpose they have

CHAPTER 6

left. Sometimes we want to get the task done quicker or we do not want to see them fail. It is important to remember that it is not about how well they do the task but that the task is fulfilling. Be sure not to take away the tasks they can still do.

A caregiver shared with me a story about her dad who was diagnosed with Alzheimer's. Dad was visiting and she was in the kitchen preparing dinner. She knew he hated to cook, but he asked how he could help. Knowing he could do the task, she gave him a potato and a peeler and turned her back on him to get back to what she was doing.

"There, I'm done!"

She turned around and saw that he had whittled the potato down to nothing and it was reduced to a pile of paper thin peels. She had a choice to correct him or give him a peacock moment.

"Wow! Dad, that is great! I never thought to do it that way. Let's make potato chips!"

A peacock moment! Great job.

CHAPTER 6
Engage

It is important to think about the word "engage" when we talk about creating purpose. I have seen this word become so popular it is often included in mission statements.

Many companies do a good job at conveying the meaning and explaining why it is so important. I would like to take this opportunity as a refresher for those who know how important engagement is, and speak to family caregivers as well who may not fully understand the "why" behind the act of engagement. In chapter 2 I talked about reaching for the brass ring of others. As a caregiver for individuals with memory loss we often find ourselves task oriented. When this occurs the person we are caring for does not feel the connection and this may result in them resisting.

We must consider successfully engaging with the person before attempting care. This allows us the opportunity to transition our connection into action.

CHAPTER 6
Jack's Connection to His Faith

Jack was a resident of a memory care neighborhood in the Midwest. The team was having challenges with Jack because he was resisting personal care and he did not like getting out of bed in the morning.

Whenever the care team would attempt to help Jack start his day he would become combative. The team tried getting him up at a different time of day to see if he preferred late morning, but to no avail. Jack would always lash out and it got to the point where the caregivers were reluctant to go in his room to help him. The director of the program contacted me and asked if I would visit and support them with Jack.

The first thing I did was work with the clinical team to find out other acute illnesses that could be causing the behavior. Jack had always been a challenge with morning care and after reviewing his case with the team we did not find any underlying medical reasons why Jack was combative. The next step was to learn about Jack, who he was, what were

CHAPTER 6

his brass rings in life, his accomplishments, his likes and dislikes, what is under his iceberg.

It is so important for family members to be actively involved regardless of what services and programs their loved ones are enrolled in. The more we know about a person, the more successful that person will be.

We did have some information about Jack in his file, but it was not enough to go on. After speaking with Jack's wife we learned that he was a very active person in his church, and since arriving at the neighborhood, he always carried a bible. Even though he was no longer able to read the bible it provided comfort to have it with him.

I asked his wife to tell me more about some of the obligations he had at church and what gave him purpose. I also asked about his routine, if he said a morning and evening prayer, or perhaps said grace at mealtime. Jack's wife said he was a member of a church prayer group many years ago but was uncertain if he continued with his morning and evening prayers since being in this community.

CHAPTER 6

After learning what was under Jack's iceberg we had a meeting with the caregivers. Mike, one of the caregivers who had frequently been on the receiving end of Jack's angry episodes, volunteered to try and get Jack ready for the day. Instead of going into Jack's room as he had done in the past, Mike would try a different, hopefully more successful approach as discussed by the group. This engagement would be an attempt to transition a connection with Jack to caregiving.

Knowing a person, learning what is under the iceberg, is so very helpful when trying to identify connections of engagement.

Mike gently knocked on Jack's door, walked into the room, and turned on a soft white light from a lamp near the window. He stood in the middle of the room with his hands wide open and his eyes closed and began to recite a morning prayer.

"Dear lord we thank you for this day. I thank you for my dear friend Jack as we say the prayer you have given us. Our father who art in heaven, hallowed be thy name." As Mike continued with the prayer he

CHAPTER 6

heard Jack's faint voice join in, reciting the prayer in a toothless mumble. Mike smiled and kept going, "Dear lord, thank you so much for this day and thank you for my friend Jack. As we rise and shine, God is good." Jack replied, "All the time!" Mike repeated, "All the time," and Jack said, "God is good."

On his own, Jack threw off the covers and sat up in bed. While he did this Mike made his way over to the window and lifted the shade. As the light poured into the room Mike stood by Jack and said, "God is good," and Jack got up out of bed and walked with Mike into the bathroom.

Jack's brass ring was going back to what he knew, what he loved, what comforted him, from one moment to the other. Jack did not remember Mike, but because he honored who Jack was, Mike made him feel that he must be a friend. We added this very important act of purpose to Jack's service plan.

We as caregivers are only as strong as our weakest link so it was important not only for Mike, but for all caregivers to have this information and to know the connection they needed to make with Jack before care.

Take a moment to think about the person you are caring for and what their brass rings are. What can you do to engage prior to supporting care tasks? What will help you and those who care for your loved one to transcend connection into care? What do you know about someone's iceberg that will help them through the day that will create acts of purpose and positive engagement.

Tom — "Get Back To Work!"

Tom was a retired construction foreman who had worked locally. He was a man's man and stood about 5 feet tall. He was happy when he had purpose, but leave him to his own devices and he was quick to create purpose, which was counterproductive for the team. When bored Tom would yell at someone to get back to work as he may have done many times while on the job.

One day I was in my office and accidentally spilled all the paper dots out of the three hole punch. They were all over the floor. The timing could not have been more perfect, as I heard Tom raising his voice at someone. I hurried out of my office and using body language as well as my voice, I told Tom I needed his help. It worked. He said, "Sure, what's wrong?" As we walked to my office, I shared that I had a mechanical malfunction and it made a mess. I explained that I had to get to a meeting and needed help so I wouldn't be late. I gave him the carpet sweeper that was in my office and showed him what happened and asked if he could take care of this for me. His exact words were, "Oh, for Christ's sake, of course I will!" and off he went sweeping the office.

This worked so well that during the times when Tom was idle we would take the three hole punch out and shake it down the hallway leaving paper dots everywhere. We didn't even need to say anything to Tom, who would already be heading for the sweeper to clean up the mess.

Purpose!

CHAPTER 6

Please note that after the act of purpose is complete, there is something very important to share with the individual that is performing the act. All acts must be accompanied with an expression of gratitude. Think about the peacock. After Tom swept the floor we would say, "Thank you so much," "You made my day," "I couldn't have had such a productive day without you."

How do you think that made Tom feel? The answer is, proud as a peacock.

Another lesson I learned is that we are quick to ask the person with memory loss a question like, "do you want to...?" that often produces the answer, "No." For example we ask, "Do you want to eat?" "Do you want to take a shower?" "Do you want to take your pills?" "Do you want to come sing some songs?" "NO!" One of the reasons why people may answer a question with the word no is because it is safe. There is nowhere to go from "No", so there are no expectations, no risk of failure.

CHAPTER 6

There are times when you want to drop your brass ring and reach for theirs, but when the answer is always the same and you are having problems motivating the individual with memory loss to even just take a walk, try using another approach.

Have you ever been asked to go somewhere because the person wanted someone to go with? Perhaps it was a place you had no intentions of ever going to; however, after you went there, you were glad you did.

"Mary, do you want to.....?"

In one community there was a resident named Mary who would often say "No" when asked to join in on a program.

During one of the team in-services on Engagement I asked how we can inspire someone to join in? There were many great answers and one that we tried that day was a success. Instead of going up to Mary and asking, "Do you want to go for a walk?" and having Mary say, "No," something else happened because of the way the caregiver inspired her. The caregiver

CHAPTER 6

walked over to Mary, got down at eye level, and first gave her a peacock moment.

"Mary, I love that color on you!" Mary smiled. The caregiver looked out the window and said, "Mary, it is a beautiful day out there." Giving Mary time to process she said, "It is?" "Oh yes, and I really want to go out and feel the warm sun on my back, but I don't want to go alone. Would you join me?" Mary thought for a moment and said, "Okay, maybe for a little while." The caregiver responded, "Oh thank you I didn't want to go alone."

This is an example of an act of purpose that was inspiring for Mary. Too often caregiving leads to checking off tasks, but it is important to see the person first.

Mary felt like she was needed and felt appreciated when she said, "yes." Try and replace the words, "Do you want to?" with the words "I would love your help."

CHAPTER 6

As we age things happen in our lives. Our children grow up and no longer need us. We retire and no longer have a job to go to. We may no longer be able to drive and go to our place of worship or visit our family and friends. Losing purpose does not happen overnight and is something we slide into. No longer having purpose slows us down mentally and physically.

The Takeaway

For home-based caregivers: Don't be afraid to give your loved ones small tasks to do. The task may need to be broken down into a simpler format. As the disease progresses, they may not do it correctly, but it is your goal to make them feel valued and proud to be contributing. Always be sure to express gratitude and thanks for their help. If they get it wrong, you just learned a valuable lesson – you won't do it again. If it doesn't work at all or they cannot do the task, don't get upset and throw in the towel, find something else they can have more success in doing.

CHAPTER 6

Think about how wonderful it is to have someone rub your back. This is something you may ask them to do for you. If they are successful, tell them by saying, "Thank you so much for my morning back rub. You have such a healing touch, it feels so nice." They will feel like they have done such a wonderful thing for you. Purpose!

For community caregivers: Too often as caregivers we are so task oriented, and even though that is important, we need to move away from the task and take a few moments to connect. The act of engagement will make the task more successful and the person you are caring for will feel loved and supported by you.

Value and empathize with those who lose purpose as they age.

CHAPTER 7
The Impact of Dementia on Sexual and Intimate Relationships

"Seniors have sex. There, I said it."
Kelly McCarthy

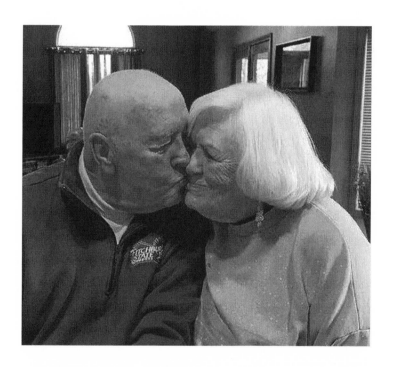

Now I bet some of you were awaiting this topic with bated breath and full of excitement, while others of you may want to skip right over it. Why is sex so taboo? Why do we squirm even more when we think about older adults having sex? The topic of sex can be uncomfortable to begin with and we all have either a cultural or personal belief system about sex and intimacy and that can weigh down the success for a proper review of the situation when caring for someone. Although there is a general gradual decline in sexual activity as we age, and there may be changes in how couples express their love for one another, it does not mean sex and intimacy is any less important. As the senior population continues to increase this is a topic that must be discussed and supported. So let's begin with discussing the difference between intimacy and sexuality.

Intimacy is a closeness, a connection to someone or something. It can be a warm friendship, a feeling of belonging, the feeling of being loved and to love others.[1]

This can be demonstrated by a friend, a relative, or a caregiver. As a caregiver please know this is very important. We're not talking about sex. You play an integral part in making someone have a sense of belonging by meeting this very important emotional core need. If a person does not feel emotionally connected, they may not be well adjusted to their surroundings.

Sexuality is an expression of interest in sex, and may involve words, gestures, or activities that attempt to display physical attraction.[2]

So, there are two different types of closeness that people enjoy. One is having that warm relationship with someone, and the other involves physical attraction.

To Love and Be Loved

Abraham Maslow proposed a theory about human needs as depicted in the pyramid on the next page.[3] We see that love, intimate relationships, and belonging are psychological needs. I am of the opinion that to love and be loved is an emotional core need.

CHAPTER 7

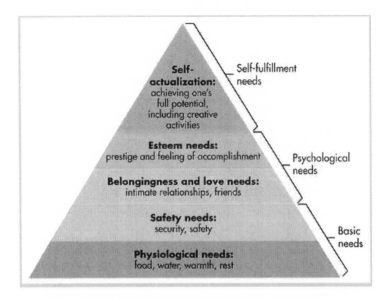

If sexuality and intimacy are so important to us as human beings, why are we not giving it enough attention when we are caring for someone who may no longer have the ability to share intimately or sexually.

If you are a partner in a relationship with someone and there is a comfortable feeling of closeness, both intimately and sexually, shared routines can be activities that attempt to display physical attraction. The activities of daily living can turn into wonderful ways of expressing love for one another. Tasks like

CHAPTER 7

applying lotion on your partner or helping to unhook a bra with a gentle rub of the back can be some of the ways to share the feelings of giving and receiving love.

Now imagine that your partner has progressive memory loss. Let's review some of the challenges both caregivers and people with memory loss can experience as the disease progresses.

- Misidentification
- Hypersexuality
- Inappropriate sexual behavior
- Judgment
- Indifference
- Medical condition

Misidentification:

This can be the most difficult challenge to face when caring for someone with memory loss. A spouse of 60 years may not recognize you, or a child may be misidentified as a husband or wife. The person may be in a second marriage, but sees the current partner as the spouse from the first marriage.

CHAPTER 7

All of these scenarios can be very difficult to face. Spouses have expressed feelings of sadness or anger thinking they have been replaced. It is important to separate the person you love from the disease.

You must be sure there is a balance between the need of the person with dementia and yourself. One of the most difficult things I have seen are spouses trying to work through transitioning themselves into whoever their loved ones believe them to be.

Some of you may remember the story of Supreme Court Justice Sandra Day O'Connor and how her husband found comfort connecting with another individual in the memory care community he resided in.[4] It took strength and understanding on Justice O'Connor's part to see beyond him as her husband, and to instead think about his personal well-being as he discovered this connection. There are no clear answers on how to work through this, but there are associations and professionals you can talk with to help you.

While traveling throughout the country, I have seen many individuals with Alzheimer's disease "lose"

CHAPTER 7

their spouse, that is, when the spouse can no longer be recognized and they vanish from the person's mind. Our brass ring is "Til death do us part." They may remember the young you, but not the old. You have spent your life with this person and the day has come when they walk into a room or wake up in the middle of the night beside you only to think you are a stranger. Try to put yourself in their shoes and imagine how that must feel. The individual with memory loss may also experience periods of lucidity when they recognize you or consider you familiar.

Be compassionate and do your best to not make it personal. The biggest pitfall with this is that the partner feels that the person with memory loss "knows better," and they are trying to "pull one over on me." This disease stinks and can be quite a roller coaster ride, so it is very important to find support. Specialized support groups such as young onset and spousal groups can be most helpful.

Hypersexuality:
While meeting with some audience members after a talk I had given, I noticed this woman who appeared to be in her 80's standing at the back of the line. She

waited for everyone to finish speaking with me before finally approaching and telling me about her husband. She said her husband was diagnosed with Alzheimer's about four years ago and she was taking care of him at home.

One of the challenges she had was that he was hypersexual. He was frequently asking her for sex and she asked me what she should do. First and foremost I would always recommend that you speak with your spouse's physician regarding the challenges surrounding sexual activity. I asked what her response to him was when he asks for sex and she said, "I make light of it and redirect him on to something else." She said he wouldn't force the issue and when she refused he would sometimes go to the basement where they had a rumpus room, turn on the TV, put a video tape in the VCR, and masturbate.

Again, and I think this is important to stress, with hypersexuality it is necessary to get a proper diagnosis, and I reminded her to have a conversation with his physician to be sure his hypersexuality was not attributed to a medical condition. There are possible treatments your doctor may recommend such as hormone therapy or other medications to regulate libido. I did mention to her that, barring any religious or cultural beliefs, masturbation is considered a natural act, and because he was still doing it in a private place and although it might be hyperactivity, it was not sexually inappropriate. She was relieved to hear this and even cracked a smile once she realized it was okay. Part of her felt like she failed as a spouse for not wanting to interact with him sexually every time he asked. Although she was going to share her husband's hypersexuality with his doctor, she did not feel like she had to do something about the behavior at the time.

Inappropriate sexual behavior:
I have found this to be the most misidentified behavior in my professional experience. For a behavior to be inappropriate for a person with memory loss you need to look at many things. The act may be appropriate, but if he/she is doing the act in public because their judgment is off, it becomes inappropriate. There may also be acts that are deemed inappropriate, but upon further review

it is discovered to be a medical condition, and the following story about Bruce is a good example of this.

Hidden Under Bruce's Iceberg

Bruce was 86 years old and had been living in the community for just under one year. One day Bruce had a behavior the team was concerned about. Bruce would pull his pants down, exposing his genital area, and ask the team members to look. He did this about three or four times and each time the caregivers would report it to the nurse. After examining Bruce, the nurse did not find any medical concerns. The nurse reviewed Bruce's medication sheet, which showed there was an order for Haldol PRN (as needed) for agitation, so he was given the pill and the reason was noted as, "due to inappropriate sexual acts."

Bruce's daughter came in to visit the next day and asked why her dad was sleepy and appeared to be drugged up. The director spoke with the daughter and explained what happened, and after hearing about the incident she talked with the director about

CHAPTER 7

her dad's medical history and the behavior surrounding it, and that he misidentified his scrotum as hemorrhoids. She mentioned that she used to tell her dad that it was a part of his body and did not need to be removed. This worked for him and he was okay with the explanation. The team looked at the history in Bruce's personal life story which provided the hemorrhoid surgery information, but not the behavior he exhibited because of it. The family thought the behavior had subsided and didn't share this information with the community. This is a great example of the Iceberg concept and highlights the point that not all things will be shared, so we need to ask the questions.

So, with the diagnosis of dementia, we sometimes throw everything in the bucket of sexually inappropriate. I'm not saying this is wrong, but it is important not to place a negative stigma on the act of sexuality. We need to investigate further to identify what the unmet need is.

CHAPTER 7

Judgment and Acts of Indifference:

As we know, Alzheimer's and other related dementias are not just about forgetfulness, they affect judgment as well. It is important to remember that although you have a relationship with your loved one, and may have for many years, you must understand that with this disease the act of sex may be very difficult for them.

Some of the challenges might be that they are no longer sexually aroused or they cannot satisfy you because they have forgotten the steps or sequences it takes to engage in sexual activity. There may also be a problem with physical touch as fine motor skills decline with this disease or they may lose their ability to connect and will come across to you as indifferent. This may not only be occurring because of the disease, but may be attributed to medications that decrease libido.

There is not a lot of information on this topic for many reasons. What is important is that the support services for families, such as home care, day care, and residential communities, should be investing in much needed education about sex and intimacy in their respective environments.

The Takeaway

For home-based caregivers: Please know how important it is to connect and be comfortable with speaking to someone regarding the challenges you are having around sexuality and intimacy. If you are a partner, know that being creative with the care tasks you provide can give you and your partner the intimacy or warm relationship you both may be in search of. Resources out there for you are:

- Psychiatrists that specialize in dementia
- Social workers within the community
- The director of the program who specializes in dementia care
- Your local Alzheimer's Association or other Alzheimer's or dementia programs in your area
- Support groups that fit your needs
- Spousal groups, which may make you feel more comfortable talking about the challenges you face with your partner

Chapter 7

For community caregivers: It is very important to understand your responsibility in protecting the vulnerable. The leadership team at your community or agency should always be aware of any sexual encounter that involves the person you are caring for. All strategies and interventions should be included in their service plan so that everyone is informed and the individuals involved are kept safe. Supporting the team when challenges like this occur is very important. Create standards and practices to identify dignity around sexuality and intimacy, which should include the LGBTQ community. You don't have to accept other's sexual lifestyle as your own: however, it is important to understand cultural or personal diversity and not judge. Also know that Alzheimer's and related dementias can affect someone's impulsivity. If you are asked for a sexual favor, under no circumstances are you to entertain the offer. Responding to sexual advances with laughter or giggling may create a read of flirtation and now the person is in the process of an active chase. More effective approaches may be to let them know you are not that kind of person and walk away if they are safe, or tell them you are going to give them some time alone and that you will return later.

CHAPTER 7

It is important for you to be properly trained on approach. Lastly, understand that those you care for still need to love and be loved. Remember this is not sex, it is the gift of a close friend. It is important that you find ways as a team to create successful means to connect with all of the individuals you care for.

Chapter 8
Communication

"We have two ears and one mouth so that we can listen twice as much as we speak" Epictetus

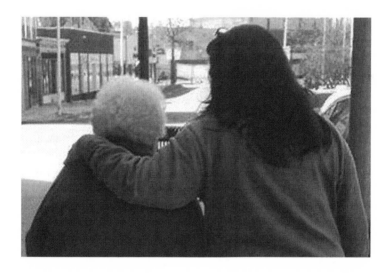

Communication is the root of all relationships and one of the most common ways we communicate is to have a conversation with one another through spoken words.

When we are caring for those with memory loss who no longer have the ability to communicate with us in the typical ways we are comfortable with, we must

Chapter 8

change the way we communicate with them. This is perhaps one of the greatest challenges caregivers are faced with as the disease progresses.

You may not always be able to set the stage when having a conversation, but you should pay attention to the following:

- The environment — Will surrounding noise be a distraction? How about lighting? Is there a glare or low lighting that may cause misidentification of people or items?

- The participants — How are we using our facial expressions, tone of voice, and body language? Does it go along with the conversation? Do we have the information that is under their iceberg, such as how they communicate? For example, if a person was in the military or law enforcement and spent their career life communicating in a direct manner, the exchange may be different than with someone who communicated in a more soft spoken, nurturing way. Is their communication influenced by cultural

CHAPTER 8

customs, such as eye contact and/or physical touch. Are you listening? Do they need time to process?

Dementias may severely impair a person's ability to communicate through words, and as this type of communication declines it can often be replaced with a "read", which is a person's interpretation of the space they are in. For example, showing someone a plate of food reinforces that they read it is time to eat. Squinting eyes and hands on hips may give them a read that is completely different than what you intend. If we do not look friendly, we are not friendly. This is why it is so important to pay particular attention to your body language when communicating with someone with memory loss.

As verbal skills decline you may find using pictures or gestures more successful, and you may also find it important to give them time to process the information they are receiving. What may seem easy for us to do is now broken into a sequence of steps for them, such as receiving, processing, and responding. Other considerations may be physical challenges, such as hearing loss, visual decline, and, more specifically with Alzheimer's, the inability to perceive depth perception and a shrinking of their peripheral vision. You need to take all of this into account when attempting to connect with the person through communication.

Unconsciously, we may fall into the trap of reflective communication and respond to someone in the manner in which they are communicating with us, for example, an angry comment begets an angry response. Instead, we must be genuinely thoughtful in the way in which we respond to them. Our goal is to convey that we care and that we value what is being communicated to us.

Milton's Need to be Heard

Milton resided in the very first memory care neighborhood I oversaw. Milton originally moved in with his wife and within three months she passed unexpectedly. Cognitively he was not able to retain the death of his wife, and although he didn't look for her on a regular basis, when he did he would repeatedly insist on her whereabouts. Milton was about 6'-5", with a sturdy build. Milton never had a physical confrontation with anyone, but his voice and size were intimidating. When Milton was angry and wanted to know where his wife was, the care team would say in passing and kept their distance, "We haven't seen her, but when we do we'll let her know you are looking for her," or they would try to redirect him by saying, "Would you like a cup of coffee?" None of this was working and one of the care team members informed me that Milton's behavior was escalating. Initially I stood outside my office and observed Milton and I could see that both fists were clenched and down by his side, he was leaning forward with one foot in front of the other, his shoulders were up, and he was very angry. As a result of my observation I knew Milton was about to blow! So, I approached him and said, "Milton, I see that you're upset and I take full responsibility. I'm sorry." I had a notepad and pen with me and as I showed them to Milton I said, "I want to write down everything that's bothering you, so let's talk." I saw an immediate physical release from Milton as he unclenched his fists and dropped his shoulders, and with a big growl shouted, "Jesus Christ, it's about time somebody listened!"

Believe me, I do not always get it right. Being mindful of your delivery can create a successful response to someone like Milton, rather than using a cookie cutter approach. Understand when things do not work and never be afraid to ask for help. This is particularly important for the home-based caregiver who is caring for a loved one on their own.

Loss of Inhibitions

The next opportunity we may find ourselves in is when the mindful approach does not work. Have you ever been in a situation where you have tried your best to communicate effectively only to have an insult thrown your way? A conversation may have personally resulted in the response, "Wow, she has a fat ass!" Or, imagine a male nurse trying to give a resident their medications and hearing, "You're a nurse? You must be a faggot."

There are two reasons why people with memory loss do this. The first reason is they have lost their inhibitions. I use the example of a venetian blind in my trainings to explain what a loss of inhibitions is. People with progressive memory loss at some point begin to lose their filter and their venetian blind may be stuck open, resulting in their thoughts coming through and being said. Traveling in airports I saw a lot of different people and I must admit I found myself thinking, "Who the hell dressed you?" I would never in a million years say what I was thinking to the person and luckily my venetian blind was working properly. Some caregivers will say to me, "Kelly, I get that their filter is gone but what they are saying is downright mean!" Which leads us to the other reason, they are a product of their environment. We are all products of our environment. How we were raised and the experiences we had in our childhood, whether good or bad, stay with us.

My daughter doesn't know where my father has been, and my father will never know where my daughter is going. Generations may not understand one another because they have not been through the social experience. They may have biases from where they grew up. It is a lifelong imprint that has been made on them.

CHAPTER 8

The following is a great little story from a friend of mine, and while journeying through her father's communication decline, she shared with me a great take away from one of her visits with him. Maureen's dad has Alzheimer's and they were sitting together talking and he asked, "How's that lady?" Maureen responded in a manner most people would and said, "What lady? Who are you talking about?" Her dad seemed to be annoyed with her questions and said, "The lady. How's the lady?" "Dad, who are you talking about? What lady? Is it someone I know?" Maureen realized right away that her responses were only frustrating her dad, so she tried communicating with him in a different way. "Oh yes, the lady! She's doing great, and the next time I see her I'll tell her you were asking for her." He snapped back, "Well Goddamnit, I knew you knew who I meant!"

This is a man who never swore a day in his life and Maureen could tell how quickly he became frustrated by her questions. By changing her approach and not needing to know everything right away, it worked. What was even better was when her dad was relaxed she was able to identify that he said the word realtor, which put the puzzle together for her and at that point she knew who he was talking about. Maureen first decreased her dad's anxiety and then began the process of figuring it out. This is a wonderful example of Maureen changing her communication approach to fit her dad's cognitive decline.

By nature we ask questions to try and understand what someone is saying. For someone with memory loss, questions may cause undue anxiety and negative feelings such as frustration and anger. We need to pay attention to the inflection of their voice, their body language, their facial expressions. Are they scared? Are they in pain? Are they excited? What can we do to ride their wave and decrease their anxiety?

My Most Rewarding Work Week

On a very cold snowy day in January, I got an early morning phone call from work, which is never good, right? Sure enough, my presence was needed immediately at a community in New Jersey. A boiler room explosion blew part of the roof off the building leaving nearly 200 residents without heat and they

CHAPTER 8

had to be evacuated. Other than the contractor, who suffered a minor injury, luckily no one else was hurt.

All air and rail travel had been suspended due to the snowstorm, so my only option was to get in my car and drive there. The trip to New Jersey would normally take about 4 hours and 40 minutes, but with the near white out conditions it took me 7 hours and 20 minutes of harrowing, white knuckled driving, at a top speed of 20 miles per hour all the way down I-95 South.

As the clock neared midnight, I finally arrived safe and sound and got right to work with the team. Together with amazing associates who worked all through the day and night, we were able to place our independent and assisted living residents in a nearby hotel, and our memory care residents were placed in a local nursing home.

The memory care residents were going to be somewhat challenged in their new surroundings due to the design and layout of the nursing home. The community these residents were coming from was specifically planned out to allow them to wander

CHAPTER 8

throughout the neighborhood. This was not the case with the nursing home, which was much smaller, but it was better than the hotel.

After very little sleep, sunrise arrived too early, but the team was ready to begin a new day and to relieve those who worked the night shift. Despite the challenges the nursing home design gave us, we were able to turn a multipurpose room into a makeshift dining area, and although the residents were free to roam, they felt more comfortable in this common space. As you entered through the French doors there were chairs lined up along the walls with two small tables in the middle of the room.

Throughout most of the day there were at least 20 residents in this space so it was difficult to do multiple programs. Nevertheless, this common area was always boisterous and full of life, and most of the residents did quite well under the circumstances.

There were some residents though that did not appreciate the cramped quarters and loud noise levels and would get overwhelmed with the extra stimulation. Relocation stress is real and the associates did very well with allowing the residents who felt overwhelmed to leave the room and go out into the hallway. This was my first time meeting some of these residents so I went around the room to introduce myself to everyone and talk with them.

Betty - "You are love."

When I met Betty she was not only challenged by the noise, she was unable to articulate her distress through words due to a mild case of aphasia.[1] Despite the challenges, Betty enjoyed being around others and preferred to stay in the room. Had this not been the case, I would have moved her into a quieter area.

Moving along down the row of chairs a few seats from where Betty was sitting, I began chatting away with another resident. While I was talking, I noticed that Betty was looking right at me and she appeared to have a disgusted look on her face.

I ended my conversation and walked over to Betty who was still staring at me and she said very clearly,

CHAPTER 8

"And you don't pay attention, so I'm not going to waste my time!" I immediately knelt down on one knee in front of her and off to the side so she wouldn't feel threatened, while maintaining eye contact, I said, "You are right and I am sorry I was not giving you my undivided attention. Do you forgive me?" Betty looked at me and said, "Well, where else am I going to go!" I laughed and that broke the ice.

The room was still quite lively and it was difficult to concentrate, but Betty did not want to return to her room. By chatting with her, I gave her something to focus on, and her anxiety and frustration with the noise slowly subsided.

A caregiver happened to walk past as Betty and I were talking, and she was dressed in a uniform. The undershirt she wore was sticking out a little, but by today's standards she was dressed very nicely.

Betty was a woman of many words and she was not afraid to use them, especially when she was angry. That's when everyone knew what she was thinking and she was proficient with using profanity. When

CHAPTER 8

Betty became emotional there was a little more clarity in her speech and as the caregiver walked by, Betty looked at me and said, "Look at the way she's dressed. I would never walk out of the house like that. She looks like a fucking slob. I always dressed up and looked my best." I placed my hands out in front of Betty, and as I continued making eye contact with her, she reached for my hands. Betty continued speaking and I was not able to catch every word, but one word I did hear clearly was poetry. I asked if she enjoyed hearing poems and she said, "Oh yes," and as she closed her eyes I could tell it was something she most certainly cherished.

Remember now, things are still a bit chaotic, there are about 25 residents sitting around in the room, and associates are changing shift. Amid the hustle and bustle I asked if she wouldn't mind me sharing a poem I wrote many years ago. I told her it was fitting with all the snow we just got. So, while on one knee at Betty's eye level and holding her hands, I began to recite my poem:

CHAPTER 8

Clean and white the ground did lay,
the sky was of the purest gray.
Trees were aged with white sideburns
of leafless wisdom winter turns.

I was very animated as I recited the poem, using facial expressions and voice inflection, and I could tell that Betty was listening intently to everything I had to give. I continued on to the last part of the poem.

Mirror images have lost their shine
to snow covered sheets of satin design
that filled the air with shining light,
to seem like day when it was night.

When I ended the poem Betty's face reddened and tears filled her eyes as she reached up and touched my face. Betty slowly said to me, "You ... are ... love," and gave me a hug.

In the midst of a loud, makeshift dining room with nowhere to go, a connection was made. This connection was a gift to me that will last as long as I am able to remember.

CHAPTER 8
Alice - "I Can't Get No Satisfaction."

Also while working the week in New Jersey, I was honored to meet Alice. She had young onset Alzheimer's with expressive aphasia,[2] so her verbal communication skills were diminished to one word, "Yes," or so we thought! She paced throughout the day and if you said, "Hi Alice," her response was always, "Yes, yes."

For the first part of the week my communication style with Alice was limited. I paid attention to her facial expressions and body language, making sure she was happy. Even though she would say "Yes," at times you could tell she meant "No." One day she had a visitor. Her brother-in-law stopped in to see how Alice was doing. He would typically come in with Alice's sister, his wife, but she was under the weather. Through talking with him, he shared with us that Alice went to every Rolling Stones concert that came to town. He said she knows every word to all the songs and can sing along. This was a wonderful example of finding out something below Alice's iceberg that we wouldn't know otherwise. So, I grabbed my cell phone and found a Rolling Stones song, "(I Can't Get No) Satisfaction," and began playing it for Alice. It was incredible! She sang every word while the team danced! It was so surprising and such an "aha" moment. We continued the rest of the week connecting with Alice by singing various Rolling Stones songs.

This was a week where I was not only a director, but I was there to be whatever the team needed me to be. It was a triage process and I got back to the basics of caregiving. The week validated why I chose this vocation. It was a week where I was able to put into practice what I teach.

Communication can be quite a challenge for many people with Alzheimer's and related dementias. When the conversation becomes difficult to follow, the goal is to listen more and talk less. Trust me when I say this is not easy for me! However, I have learned that the more I listen to all the words, even if they are not in the right order when spoken, the more successful the conversation will be. Instead of asking a bunch of questions to try and untangle a mishmash of words, try listening and pick up on the words that have emotions tied to them. Betty said,

CHAPTER 8

"Oh yes!" and as she closed her eyes I could tell it was something she most certainly cherished.

The Takeaway

For home-based caregivers: Some family members and friends may find it difficult to visit a loved one with memory loss when they are no longer able to communicate in the way we are familiar with. I have on occasion heard family members tell me it is difficult to see the person as they are now, or "What's the point? They're not going to remember anyway."

I will never judge anyone for the decisions they make about visiting people: however, I will do my best to inspire you to enter the room. Your loved one is still there. You can communicate with people in ways other than speech, such as touch or your smile. I understand the difficulty for some of you to visit a loved one who has changed so much. For a moment place yourself in their shoes and know that it can be very lonely without you.

Chapter 8

For community caregivers: You are only as strong as the weakest link in your community/organization. If there is valuable information about ways to communicate or interventions that create successful outcomes for the person you are caring for, everyone needs to know about them. This information needs to be on their service plan.

This is a perfect example of "You're not just a ..." You're not just a maintenance person, a caregiver, a programming person. Often times you are everything to the person you are caring for, to their family, and to the company you work for.

CHAPTER 9
I Want to Go Home

"I want this checkered tablecloth when you pass on.
It reminds me of home. We have had it forever and I
want to remember."
My son, George Silvia III

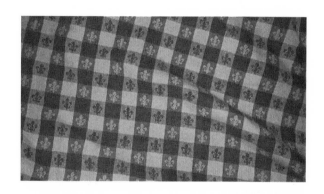

"I want to go home!" Have you ever had this said to
you by someone you were caring for? Whether the
individual challenged with progressive memory loss
is living at home, living with a family member, or
living in a residential community, these words have
often been said. So, what do they mean? Caregivers
are quick to ask, "Where is home?" or "Who is
there?" They may even tell the person with memory
loss, "You are home." As you can imagine you may

CHAPTER 9

be in for trouble and I would instead ask that you remember the peacock moment and ask yourself what the individual's brass ring is.

When you have a busy day that is full of stress, excitement, and physical activity, and it runs into the evening hours, how do you feel when you finally arrive home? Do words like relief, relaxed, safe, secure, and loved come to mind? If they do, you are not alone. It stands to reason that home is not only a place, but also a feeling.

Take a few minutes to think about some of the things that make you feel like you are "home." The granny afghan my nana made me that is hanging over the back of my rocking chair makes me feel at "home." The blue checkered tablecloth my son loves, and the coasters I strongly demand everyone use when visiting my house, make me feel at "home." And let's not forget that my favorite soap, the pink pill shaped bar with the imprint of a bird on one side, makes me feel "home." Hotels are a part of my life and I don't bring my favorite soap along with me. Even though these hotels are a makeshift home

CHAPTER 9

while I'm on the road, I love the feeling of home when I use my pink bar of soap — I'm "home."

All of the things we feel can create a sense of "home." As mentioned in chapter 7, it is important to remember the person's emotional core needs to love and be loved, to belong, and to feel like themselves. These things are extremely important to everyone.

Do you see why it can be especially important to those with memory loss? Their brass ring is the feeling of home. What do you know about the person you are caring for to make them feel safe, loved, secure, and connected? If a person with memory loss doesn't feel at "home," who is responsible for getting them there? If you said, "we are," that would be correct.

Let's get back to being in the moment. Someone looks at you and says, "I want to go home." You as the caregiver do not have the time at that given moment to do the research you need to help you understand what home is. So now what do you do? What can you say to maintain a person's dignity,

CHAPTER 9

show them you care, and value their emotional state while redirecting them away from their repeated insistence on going home?

In order for you to maintain a person's dignity you need to be on the same page with them, meaning that you understand their emotional need at that moment. Do they have a sense of urgency? Are they scared, lonely, or feeling bored? These emotions may need a different redirect to be successful. For example, if a person is stating, "I want to go home" with a persistent sense of urgency, we most likely will not be successful using statements like, "Well, let's get a cookie!", or "Want to go sing a song?", or "Want to go watch TV with me?"

The person with memory loss most likely will not feel connected because their sense of urgency is not valued. The key is to know a person, know what is under their iceberg that can assist you in valuing him or her. Instead of asking a question like, "Where's home?", you may want to hone in on the person's facial expressions and body language, their tone of voice and inflection, then show them in your eyes that you care about what they are saying.

CHAPTER 9

Create your own sense of urgency that may touch upon something they value. The next story is a great example of this.

Millie the Cat Lover

Millie was a woman who was a day stay in one of our assisted living communities. She lived with her daughter who worked weekdays, and because she was not able to be home alone, Millie went to our adult day care program five days a week. This gave her daughter peace of mind.

For the most part, Millie enjoyed participating in the day program; however, every once in awhile she would want to go home and did not understand that she needed to wait for the afternoon when the van would come to take her and the others home. Many times they were able to successfully redirect Millie's repetitive thoughts about going home with programs that were happening at that moment. There were times the team needed to be more creative with their redirect. Millie was an individual who was a bit more advanced with the progression of Alzheimer's. Her sense of reasoning had diminished and she relied heavily on reads. The cues she got either helped or hindered the redirect away from wanting to go home.

We discovered that underneath Millie's iceberg, she was a diehard feline lover. She would routinely converse about the many tricks she taught her cats through the years. One of the best stories she repeated was that of teaching two of her cats to use the house toilet. She had everyone at the program in hysterics when she would tell the story of how she trained them. Because of Millie's love for and connection with cats the director of the program created a cat book with pictures she pulled off the internet. In the book were cats of all breeds, domestic short hair, domestic long hair, double pawed, and yes, even a feline using the facilities! One day they found this book to be extremely helpful when Millie was looking to go home. This was turning out to be one of those days when their attempts at a redirect was not working, that is until caregiver Linda had a peacock moment idea.

Linda spotted Millie pacing anxiously around the exit doors and it was only 1:00 PM. The program

CHAPTER 9

was running a bit behind and was being delayed for about another 15 minutes. Linda took a chance and grabbed the cat book and walked over to Millie and said, "Millie, thank goodness I found you!" Linda not only said these words but showed emotion, a sense of urgency. Millie picked up on this and showed concern. "What is the matter?" Millie asked. Linda continued maintaining her sense of urgency and said, "I was wondering if you would help me before you go. My daughter's birthday is this week and she wants a cat. I don't know the first thing about cats and heard you would be a great person to talk with."

As Millie's peacock feathers were opening, Linda showed Millie the cat book. Linda also knew Millie did not like long haired cats because of the mess they made when shedding. Every time Millie talked about her love for cats, she brought up her disdain for long haired cats. It was the button that if pushed, would get Millie started, not in a bad way, but she would be emotionally sparked into a passionate conversation about cats. Of course when Linda said she was considering a long haired domestic breed, Millie's response was one with conviction. As the conversation blossomed, Linda placed her hand on Millie's back and began walking her to a nearby chair. While the conversation continued, Millie took her coat and hat off, and while looking at the pictures, strongly suggested another breed to Linda.

Using words like, "Would you help me?" is a good example of giving purpose. Saying "Before you go" does not cut the person off like it does if you say "You can't go" or "You live here now" which can cause great upset or feelings of despair. Knowing Millie's love for cats allowed Linda to connect. Furthermore, using her daughter's birthday created a sense of importance to Millie's purpose.

As I have stated numerous times before, there are no magic wands and each person is different. Know that you may not always get it right. Knowing what is under the person's iceberg along with having a goal to create a peacock moment is the best way to go. As always, the safety of the person and others is priority. If you feel you are in an unsafe situation with someone, and you are at a loss regarding what to do, call in other services to assist, such as a colleague, family member, or 911. Be sure to do it!

Chapter 9
The Takeaway

For home-based caregivers: This past story about Millie shows the importance of you sharing your loved one's social history with each support system you rely on. The more information shared that creates an emotional connection may assist your resources in providing familiar and successful redirections.

For community caregivers: I bet many of you working in residential memory care neighborhoods have heard the words, "I want to go home" from some of the people you care for. When you understand that home is not only a place, but a feeling, you will be able to begin to ask yourself the question, "What does home feel like for this person?" Using family as a resource will help you learn what the person you are caring for had in their home that will make them feel connected to their new surroundings to make it feel like home. Please try the following exercise — Walk around your house and look at what surrounds you. Identify how you feel, what stories unfold. Pay attention to the small things, like your favorite coffee mug or a

Chapter 9

handed down antique lamp. Now imagine you move into a smaller space and none of your items come with you. How would you feel if the things that once felt like home, no longer existed?

CHAPTER 10
Behaviors

"I thank God for behaviors, because if we didn't
have behaviors we may not know what the person is
trying to tell us."
Sharon Roth Maguire

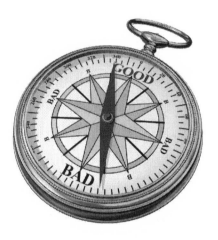

So, what is a behavior? What do you think of when
you hear the word behavior? Like many, you may
think it has a negative connotation. The truth is, if
we step back and think about it, a behavior can be
either good or bad.

CHAPTER 10

My goal in this chapter is for you to have the tools you will need to work through challenging behaviors and to work through them by creating solid interventions and not just reaching for a pill, such as an antipsychotic or anti-anxiety medication to fix it. This is not to say medications like these are not a good option, but I do believe they are not always a good first option. Behaviors are unique to each individual. Some require more detective work than others, and a physician should always be informed of any changes in behavior with the person you are caring for. It is important to rule out any medical conditions, such as a urinary tract infection, dehydration, malnutrition, medication interactions, to name a few, which may cause someone to have challenging or atypical behaviors.

As defined, a behavior is the way in which a person acts in response to a particular situation or stimulus.[1] Now that we have defined what a behavior is, let's talk about the ways to help you develop confidence in identifying successful interventions. The following are the steps I use to support communities and families in working through behaviors.

146

CHAPTER 10

Keep an Open Mind — Breathe ... and then ask yourself if it is a behavior we even need to address? If it is just different and is not causing harm, we should perhaps think more about peacock moments rather than having them conform to the norm. If we need to create interventions for a particular behavior, we must first be open-minded to understanding what they are trying to tell us, because we can only manage it once we have a full understanding of the why behind the behavior.

Teamwork/Resources — Whether you are a home-based caregiver or a community caregiver, you should have a team approach. For communities your front line team members are so valuable, and they are in fact where the rubber meets the road and have lots of information. For home-based caregivers, talk with family members and share the challenge that is happening. Be sure to include the person's life story as one of your resources in uncovering the unmet need. This is where you may want to review what is under the person's iceberg, for example, habits, what gives them purpose, and what frightens them, are just a few of the things that

CHAPTER 10

may need to be considered in working through behaviors.

You may also find support in your local Alzheimer's organizations. We are more likely to be successful in solving problems when there are multiple viewpoints involved in the process. I traveled by plane every week, but even when I landed I still had a vantage point of 10,000 feet. Have you ever been far enough away from something that you were able to see things more clearly? Having outside resources assist you in working through interventions can be a great resource. When you are too close to the situation, you may become stuck and feel limited in being able to create interventions.

A pitfall may be that the caregiver gives up — "I can't change someone's behavior!" You're right, you cannot change someone's behavior, but that does not mean you should give up. Heck, the only person's behavior we can change is our own and I don't even do that very well or I'd be a size 6! Your goal is to try to identify what they are trying to tell us. The other advantage of having an outside resource is that they may have a wide range of experiences and may have supported behaviors similar to the ones you are working through.

Collaborative Detective Work — Some people are ambitious and like to start out right away coming up with possible solutions. While some behaviors may be easy to understand the why behind the behavior, others may not. May I encourage you to not always jump to conclusions and instead start by asking questions. Be the detective. Your goal is to uncover what may be going on with the person. One of the most important indicators to check for is the person's comfort level. If the person you are caring for is not able to express to you that they are in pain, you should ask yourself what could be making him/her uncomfortable. It is also helpful to look under the person's iceberg and also go through each of the following four factors to identify possible causes:

1. Physical — Is there a physical cause? Are they in pain or have discomfort? Could the person have an infection? Some common examples are; chronic pain, fatigue, water retention, dehydration, urinary tract infection,

constipation, undiagnosed fractures, depression.

2. Environmental — Is it too hot? Too cold? Too loud? Too dark?

3. Caregiver — Is it our body language? The tone of voice? Facial expressions? Do we resemble someone they may know?

4. Psychosocial — Are they anxious or frightened? Do they have something going on that is causing them internal stress? Some common examples are nightmares, feeling privacy is being invaded, feeling neglected or abused.

Setting up a List of Possible Interventions — Once you have gone through a person's life story and the four factors, now the goal is to work on identifying the unmet need. This is where you may bullet point the things you want to implement. Don't worry about having too many or too few possible interventions. This process is intended to help you narrow down solutions to the challenging behavior.

CHAPTER 10

Follow-up and Regroup — This is where you put your bulleted interventions into action to see if they work. Interventions are rewarding but are real work. It is very easy to ask the doctor for a pill to fix something. How many of you in senior care have heard, "Do we have anything for this person?" If so, you know that the person is asking for a pill, possibly an antipsychotic or an antidepressant, which can mask the behavior, but not necessarily uncover the why behind the behavior.

It is more important to work with the doctor and others and take the time to learn who the person is, what it is that may be affecting them, what behaviors or habits they had in the past, and what interventions can be used, both pharmacological and non-pharmacological.

Don't be discouraged if you come up short and the behaviors still exist. You may need to regroup a few times to tweak what you are looking at in coming up with additional interventions.

Chapter 10
Arthur - "Shower? I already took one."

How many of you have had challenges with someone you are caring for not wanting to take a shower? Do you consider that a behavior? I have found this to be one of the most challenging behaviors caregivers have shared with me. So, let's go through the above steps in uncovering the unmet need around taking a shower with our friend Arthur.

Arthur is a 79 year old man who lives with his wife Fran and she is having a difficult time getting him to take a shower. When she asks him to take a shower he says, "No I don't want to, I already took one," or that he hasn't done anything to get dirty. Because of his response, Fran gets angry and frustrated with this recent challenge and tries to shame him into taking a shower by telling him he stinks and that he didn't take one already and that he keeps forgetting. As a result, Arthur becomes agitated and digs his heels in even more, so now Fran comes to us with this behavior.

Let's take the above example and begin the process of uncovering the why behind the behavior.

CHAPTER 10

Keep an Open Mind — Is it a behavior we even need to address? Yes, but let's be open-minded. Getting him clean does not mean he has to take an actual shower. That will be our goal, but if we have to figure out an alternative way to wash him, let's consider that a win.

Teamwork/Resources — After speaking with Fran, her resources are: her son, who lives next door; Arthur's physician; their daughter, who lives far away. Fran and her children decide to have a meeting.

Collaborative Detective Work — During the family meeting, they talk about dad's history with bathing. Through discussions and the act of reminiscing this allows them to dive deep into what is under dad's iceberg. They talk about dad's past habits in the shower. The daughter remembers always seeing a toothbrush in the shower and asks her mom if he still brushes his teeth there. They remember his favorite soap and ask if he still uses it. They remember that dad loved to sing in the shower and how embarrassed they would be if they had a

CHAPTER 10

friend over and dad was belting out, "That's Amore!"

The next step is they reviewed the four factors.

Physical — Arthur has arthritis and does not have full range of motion in his legs due to stiffness and pain. He has a difficult time with depth perception especially when colors are similar.

Environmental — The bathroom is cold until the shower is on. There is a small lip when entering the shower. The shower chair and the shower stall are both white.

Caregiver — Fran can become angry and frustrated. There are times when Arthur does not recognize Fran as his wife. Arthur is more comfortable with his son and is more successful showering when his son is there.

Psychosocial — Arthur is agitated with the way Fran communicates with him. There are times he feels his privacy is being invaded when he does not recognize Fran.

CHAPTER 10

Setting up a List of Possible Interventions — What did we learn? Did you come up with the same things Arthur's family did?

Are the items familiar to Arthur from his past being used, such as his favorite soap or a toothbrush in the shower? No, they were not. Over time Fran replaced his soap with hers and his toothbrush was now in a cup on the vanity. How about singing his favorite song? Do you think that would make an impact? Fran was so task oriented when she finally did get Arthur into the shower, the last thing she felt like doing was singing.

The interventions to put in place from what Arthur's family knows about him:

- Fran will make sure she buys his favorite soap.
- Before getting Arthur into the shower, Fran will make sure his toothbrush and toothpaste are in the shower.
- Singing Arthur's familiar song prior to getting him into the bathroom may be a possible unconscious cue for Arthur, rather than asking him, "Do you want to take a shower?"

CHAPTER 10

Physical Intervention — We know Arthur is challenged physically with arthritis. One intervention is to reach out to the doctor to consult possible over-the-counter medications prior to getting Arthur into the shower.

Environmental Intervention — Turn the shower on prior to Arthur entering the bathroom and getting him undressed. Hopefully the pill for the arthritis will make it easier for Arthur to get over the shower threshold. To create a contrast between the shower and the chair, they came up with putting a bright blue towel on the shower chair, which gave Arthur a clear target for him to sit down on. This will also help as he will not be sitting on a cold, plastic chair.

Caregiver Intervention — The family decided to have the son assist with the shower as Arthur seems to be more comfortable with a male.

Psychosocial Intervention — Arthur's son has volunteered to routinely give his dad a shower. When his son gives him a shower, he begins the process with singing his favorite song. Because the son has been successful, this eliminates Fran's stress of completing the task. Arthur's psychosocial needs are being supported by the son in maintaining his father's dignity and bringing back his familiar routine.

Follow-up and Regroup — This is where the family will talk about the interventions they have put in place. What worked and what didn't work? What needs to be tweaked?

The following is a good example of a habit found under the iceberg that can cause a behavior.

Where's My Polly

During my trainings I sometimes navigate through the room asking people in a firm voice, "Where's my polly?" Usually I get a sort of befuddled look back, then I'll ask the group, "What am I looking for?" The audience responds asking, "Is it a bird?, a dog?, a boyfriend?" As I continue to play along, now I continually become more agitated. I tell them that my next behavior is that I am beginning to disrobe. I continue to walk around the room with more anger than before asking for my polly. More than once I have had a caregiver in the audience say she is being sexually inappropriate and we need to call the nurse for medication.

I ask the group, "What do you do?" The hands go up and the resounding answer is, call the family and ask them what or who is polly. I continue with the scenario and tell them, okay, we spoke with the daughter and she says, "Oh she hasn't needed that in years." We ask her to tell us more. When the daughter was 3 years old, she often saw a hair tie on her mother's wrist and named it a polly, so the name stuck. The daughter added that mom would use her polly when she wanted to get her hair out of her eyes or when she was feeling hot.

I asked the group, "So, what am I trying to tell you?" They replied, "You're feeling hot." Exactly! It all makes sense now, doesn't it? I want the polly because I have always tied up my hair when I am feeling too hot. Habit! This is a great example of a habit. Even though my hair may be short now, it is something I had always done in the past. The behavior of taking off my clothes further confirms

CHAPTER 10

that I am feeling too hot, and because my judgment is off, I don't know how to express my need to cool off other than referring to my habit of putting my hair up with a polly.

Understanding the why behind the behavior will help you create interventions. For me, it may be getting a glass of water, opening a window, or taking off my sweater. The underlying problem was simply that I was hot. This is a good example of how we cannot control a person's behavior, but you can have a good chance of managing it once you understand the why behind it.

Do some detective work and keep asking questions to primary caregivers to learn more about what it is the person with memory loss may actually be saying. To the team, look within yourself for a moment and identify what you do or say in the privacy of your own home that can be misconstrued if you think that everyone knows what you are talking about.

CHAPTER 10
When You Feel You Are in Danger

Although we are aware that behaviors may be good or bad, it is important to note that when the person with memory loss is placing themselves or others at risk for serious injury or even death, immediate action must take place. Safeguarding the home and yourself from someone with aggressive behaviors is very important. The following are suggestions to protect those who may find themselves in a potentially dangerous situation:

1. Remove or secure firearms.
2. Lock up sharps such as knives and scissors in a safe and secure place.
3. Remove all objects in the home that could be or have been used in the past as weapons.
4. Give and show a sincere apology when an aggressive moment happens.
5. If you are aware there is pet abuse taking place, remove the animal from the environment.
6. If there are others who may potentially be in harm's way, remove them from the area and

away from the person who is showing aggressive behavior.

7. If you feel you are in danger, it is very important to have a safe place to retreat to within the home. Be sure the door has a lock and that you have access to a phone if you need to call 911.

We as caregivers are not invisible to the possible distortion and anger of an individual with Alzheimer's or related dementias. Be sure that all supporting caregivers for this person are aware of the potential for aggression as well as the possible triggers and interventions. Also, you may want to consider reaching out to your local authorities/public safety department to inquire about any alert systems they may have in place to inform them and make them aware of the situation at home.

It is important for you to know that you are not alone. Please refer to the resources section at the end of the book which identifies some support organizations that may be able to assist you.

CHAPTER 10
Wandering

Six out of every ten individuals with Alzheimer's and related dementias wander.[2]

It is important to take a few moments and review the dangers and support systems out there that can assist the caregivers in keeping the person they are caring for safe.

By itself, the act of wandering may not be dangerous. However, wandering does become a serious safety issue when the person's judgment is off, and/or they forget where they are or why they are in a particular place.

Wandering can occur in many stages of the disease, and while explaining this, let's break down two common categories of wandering:

- Wandering with Intent
- Wandering without Intent.

CHAPTER 10

Wandering with Intent: When a person has an agenda. The person may or may not have a judgment deficit at this point, but can still be challenged with the dangers of wandering.

Let's take the person who is in the early stages of the disease who starts off by walking to their local convenience store. Now, imagine that when the person starts on the intended walk there is construction going on that makes them have to go another way. The detoured route is unfamiliar and this can throw the person off course. This example is not about the person's judgment being off, but about forgetting where they are. This can add anxiety and confusion into the mix.

Another example of wandering with intent, but this time with judgment being a challenge, is that the person may be wandering in search of the bathroom. They may open a door to another space and because they have the urge to void and their judgment is off, they may very well use the space as the bathroom. It is important to note that when this happens you should not confront them. Many individuals will not remember what they did and may even think you are crazy for even considering the idea. This is not because they are lying, but in fact know at that moment that the space is not a bathroom and would never consider doing such a thing. You are not going to praise them for using the space as a bathroom, but neither should you shame them for the incident. Asking the person why they did the action may cause them upset. Try to identify the why behind the action by working through the four possible factors; Physical, Environmental, Caregivers Cause, or Psychosocial.

Wandering Without Intent: When a person is wandering without an agenda or purpose. This type of wandering often occurs in the moderate to later stages of the disease. For example, a person may touch every door handle but has no intentions of opening the door. You may want to ask yourself, "Is the person's intent being masked by the disease?" In other words, is there a reason for the wandering? Is the person thirsty, hungry, or in need of the bathroom?

This is not to say there has to be an agenda. It is ok for the person with memory loss to safely wander as

Chapter 10

long as the person is not in distress or in any danger while doing so. We as caregivers must be vigilant when allowing someone to safely wander by keeping them in our sight, as circumstances can change moment to moment.

It is important to note that just because the person in your care is not currently wandering, they may become a wanderer. If you are not set up for a safe wandering experience, the following are a few suggestions that have supported others:

- MedicAlert* & Alzheimer's Association Safe Return* — a 24 hour nationwide emergency response service for individuals with Alzheimer's or a related dementia who wander or have a medical emergency. They provide 24 hour assistance no matter when or where the person is reported missing. Read more at: http://www.alz.org/care/dementia-medic-ale rt-safe-return.asp#ixzz4V6jYGTx8
- Your local authorities — call and ask your local police and fire departments if they have a program that supports at risk individuals who may wander.

- Door and window alarms — you may want to consider installing alarm indicators. Your local hardware or electronic store will have options and prices for you to consider.
- Tracking devices — There are many different kinds. Many work on Bluetooth and have an app for your cell phone or computer which tracks the whereabouts of a certain item someone is carrying like a wallet or cell phone. Some devices can even be sewn into a coat or other article of clothing that a person wears. You can either check with your local electronic store or search online for tracking devices for people and things. You will surely come up with options to consider.

The Takeaway

For home-based caregivers: Chapter 1 talks about taking care of yourself, and the behaviors we talk about in this chapter can be some of the most stressful for you. If you begin to see challenging behaviors at home, you need to work with your resources. They are out there and you are not alone. It is best to have your resources in place ahead of

CHAPTER 10

time to have a support network for your well-being and for the person you are caring for. Some resources may be family, friends, neighbors, faith-based organizations, an Alzheimer's Association, or other related dementia organizations.

For community caregivers: When working in a community/organization it may be challenging when a behavior arises. Don't be complacent, ask for help.

It is easy to quickly ask for medication like an antipsychotic to mask a behavior, so instead, first use all of your resources, such as a physician, family, and outside resources as well as your regional team, especially those who give you a 10,000 feet vantage point. They will help you to think outside of the box to try new interventions.

Chapter 11

What Do You Do When You Don't Get It Right?

"If you are discouraged, it is a sign of pride because it shows you trust in your own power"
Mother Teresa

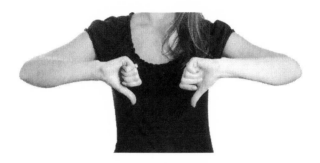

Breathe, and reread Chapter 1.

CHAPTER 12
Putting It All Together

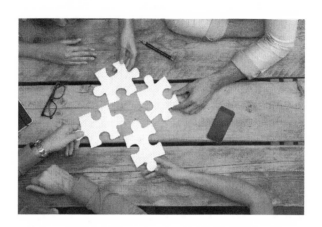

None of us are excused from the fast-paced world we live in. We are often rushed in accomplishing our daily tasks. As you may know, caring for someone with memory loss can be extremely trying when we do not slow down. Whether I am working with individuals who are caring for loved ones at home, or employees in a community or agency setting, I find it very important to be vigilant in teaching the act of appreciating a moment, that is, to step back, stop, listen, and learn.

Trying to rush memory care tasks usually results in failure for you and the person you are caring for.

CHAPTER 12

The good news is, whether you are rushing or just made a mistake on a good attempt at connecting, your failures can be as important as each success if you learn from them.

Remember, there is no magic wand, no magic approach, and most importantly, no magic pill. Some approaches will work and some will not. The key is to not beat yourself up or become so frustrated with the person you are caring for that you both become ticking time bombs ready to blow! Just breathe.

The terms I use such as, "reaching for the brass ring," "identifying what is under the iceberg," and "creating peacock moments," are methodologies that will guide you each and every moment and beyond. Using these concepts will support you in this fast-paced world to identify good outcomes in caring for and communicating with someone who has memory loss.

What is so wonderful about these three phrases is they can work, no matter what stage a person is in with memory loss. They will help you create a plan

Chapter 12

and an outlook on what may work, and to become reflective when it does not. You will not always get it right, and that's ok.

"You are not 'just a'....."

I will leave you with this one last story.

Let's go back to the New Jersey trip where the community residents were evacuated. For the residents placed in the hotel, they had challenges from their environment as well, and one of those challenges was the hotel toilet seats were too low. The evacuation happened so swiftly that there was not enough time or space to take everything that was needed, such as toilet risers.

While sitting at a triage table one evening with the team, I looked up and noticed a young businessman looking over at us. He was a very tall, handsome man, with a close shaven beard. I guessed that he was not yet thirty years old. As he slowly walked over to our table, I said to him, "Not your typical business week!" He said, "Yes, I thought it was a convention when I saw all the walkers, but I soon

CHAPTER 12

realized it was something else." We chuckled and he continued, "I remember you." "Me?" I replied. "Yes, the night I checked in, you were here in the lobby."

I could tell he had something he wanted to say, and after I explained the reason for all the walkers due to the emergency evacuation of the assisted living community, he told me this wonderful story.

"You may have heard this already, but the night I checked into the hotel and arrived at my room, an elderly lady peered out of her door from across the hall and asked for help. She seemed very worried and anxious. She said her roommate needed some help. I asked her if she wanted me to call someone and she said, 'No! It is too embarrassing.' She went on to explain how they were displaced tonight and were not used to the low toilets, and her roommate just needed help off the toilet and it should only take a minute. I thought about things for just a second, wondering what to do. My uneasiness with the situation quickly faded and I walked in the bathroom, held out my hands, and as the lady held on tight, I lifted her off the toilet. She thanked me and I walked out."

CHAPTER 12

When he finished his story, I looked at my colleague and we both had expressions of amazement on our faces. I asked him, "What is your name sir?" He smiled and replied, "My name is Alan." I said, "Alan, do you know you are a godsend?" He smiled again and said, "No, I'm just a grandson and she needed help." I thanked him for his kindness and said, "You are not 'just a' anything. At that moment for those two women you were everything." I thanked him again and said, "I wish there were more grandsons like you."

May we be blessed to know, and to be the Alan we met that night.

About the Author

Kelly has been in the senior health industry for over 20 years.

She graduated from Emmanuel College in Boston with a B.S. in Psychology and a concentration in Gerontology Rehabilitation/Management.

Kelly is a Licensed Nursing Home Administrator and Certified Dementia Practitioner. She is also a BC-DEd Board Certified Dementia Educator for NIDE National Institute for Dementia Education.

She is currently the Corporate Director of Memory Care and Resident Engagement at LCB Senior Living.

She is certified as a Master Trainer for the RI/NH/MA Alzheimer's Association Train The Trainer Memory Care state recognized training program for caregivers.

Kelly was the keynote speaker at the 2016 Alzheimer's Caregiver Conference.

Kelly holds a certificate as an Alzheimer's support group facilitator and is an Alzheimer's speaker's bureau lecturer.

While with Senior Lifestyle she has received the 2013 National ALFA Best of the Best Award for developing the "Walk With Me Program — a journey that moves us all" in the category of Supporting Families of Residents During Transitional Times.

Kelly continues to provide countrywide training and support in memory care for organizations such as the Alzheimer's Association, Memory Care Forum, and other organizations supporting individuals challenged with memory loss and their caregivers. Topics include, but are not limited to, Assisting Families with Caregiver Stress, Hiring Training and Retaining Great Care Teams, Creating a Successful Memory Care Environment, Intimacy Sexuality and Memory Care.

Kelly provides consulting and training through her company, Brass Ring Wellness, LLC.

Endnotes

Chapter 1

1. Schulz R, Beach SR. Caregiving as a Risk Factor for Mortality:
   The Caregiver Health Effects Study. JAMA. 1999;282(23):2215-2219. doi:10.1001/jama.282.23.2215.
2. The term "geriatric fiblet" was coined at the 2000 World Alzheimer's Congress as "necessary white lies to redirect loved ones or discourage them from detrimental behavior." https://www.caring.com/articles/alzheimers -code-of-ethics

Chapter 2

1. http://carousels.org/USACensus/stdqueries/c ensus-awards.html#RINGS

Chapter 3

1. Sudden Infant Death Syndrome (SIDS) - Sudden infant death syndrome (SIDS) is the unexplained death, usually during sleep, of a seemingly healthy baby less than a year old. SIDS is sometimes known as crib death because the infants often die in their cribs.

Although the cause is unknown, it appears that SIDS may be associated with abnormalities in the portion of an infant's brain that controls breathing and arousal from sleep.

Researchers have discovered some factors that may put babies at extra risk. They've also identified some measures you can take to help protect your child from SIDS. Perhaps the most important measure is placing your baby on his or her back to sleep.
http://www.mayoclinic.org/diseases-conditions/sudden-infant-death-syndrome/basics/definition/con-20020269
2. Global Deterioration Scale -
https://www.dementiacarecentral.com/aboutdementia/facts/stages/

Chapter 5
1. Dementia as symptom -
http://www.alz.org/what-is-dementia.asp
https://www.gmeded.com/gme-info-graphics/what-dementia
2. Dementia -

http://www.alz.org/what-is-dementia.asp#de
mentia
3. Alzheimer's -
   https://www.nia.nih.gov/alzheimers/topics/al
   zheimers-basics
4. Alzheimer's -
   http://www.alz.org/alzheimers_disease_what
   _is_alzheimers.asp
5. Delirium-
   http://www.mayoclinic.org/diseases-conditio
   ns/delirium/basics/definition/con-20033982

Chapter 7
   1. Intimacy -
2. a close, familiar, and usually affectionate or loving
personal relationship with another person or group.
http://www.dictionary.com/browse/intimacy
   2. Sexuality -
recognition of or emphasis upon sexual matters.
http://www.dictionary.com/browse/sexuality?s=t
   3. Maslow-
       http://www.simplypsychology.org/maslow.ht
       ml

4. O'Connor-
https://www.caring.com/articles/sandra-day-
oconnor-interview-alzheimers

Chapter 8

1. Aphasia - is an impairment of language,
affecting the   production or comprehension
of speech and the   ability to read or write.
http://www.aphasia.org/aphasia-definitions/
2. Expressive Aphasia-
http://www.aphasia.org/aphasia-definitions/

Chapter 10

1. Behavior-
https://en.oxforddictionaries.com/definition/
behaviour
2. Wandering -
http://www.alz.org/search/results.asp?q=wa
ndering&as_dt=i#gsc.tab=o&gsc.q=wanderin
g&gsc.page=1

Resources

Alzheimer's Association
225 N Michigan Ave
Chicago, IL 60611-7633
24/7 Helpline 1-800-272-3900
www.alz.org

Alzheimer's Foundation of America
322 Eighth Avenue, 7th floor
New York, NY 10001
Helpline 1-866-232-8484
www.alzfdn.org

Alzheimer's Disease Education and Referral (ADEAR) Center
800-438-4380
https://www.nia.nih.gov/alzheimers

The Association for Frontotemporal Degeneration
Radnor Station Building 2, Suite 320
290 Kings of Prussia Road
Radnor, PA 19087
267-514-7221 or 866-507-7222
www.theaftd.org

Family Caregiver Alliance
235 Montgomery Street, Suite 950
San Francisco, CA 94104
415-434-3388 or 800-445-8106
www.caregiver

Lewy Body Dementia Association
912 Killian Hill Road S.W.
Lilburn, GA 30047
LBD Caregiver: 800-539-9767
National Office 404-935-6444
www.lbda.org

MedicAlert Foundation
5226 Pirrone Court
Salida, CA 95368
1-800-432.5378
www.medicalert.org

Alzheimer's Association Facts and Figures
http://www.alz.org/facts

Made in the USA
Middletown, DE
14 February 2019